Quick Questions in
Ankle Sprains

Expert Advice in Sports Medicine

Editors

Patrick O. McKeon, PhD, ATC, CSCS
Assistant Professor
Department of Exercise & Sports Sciences
Ithaca College
Ithaca, New York

Erik A. Wikstrom, PhD, ATC, FACSM
Associate Professor
Department of Kinesiology
University of North Carolina at Charlotte
Charlotte, North Carolina

Series Editor

Eric L. Sauers, PhD, ATC, FNATA
Professor and Chair
Department of Interdisciplinary He⸺
Arizona School of Health Sci⸺
A.T. Still University
Mesa, Arizona

SLACK
I N C O R P O R A T E D

www.Healio.com/books

ISBN: 978-1-61711-817-3

Published by: SLACK Incorporated
                       6900 Grove Road
                       Thorofare, NJ 08086 USA
                       Telephone: 856-848-1000
                       Fax: 856-848-6091
                       www.Healio.com/books

Contact SLACK Incorporated for more information about other books in this field or about the availability of our books from distributors outside the United States.

Library of Congress Cataloging-in-Publication Data

Quick questions in ankle sprains : expert advice in sports medicine / editors, Patrick O. McKeon, Erik Wikstrom.
   p. ; cm.
 Includes bibliographical references and index.
 ISBN 978-1-61711-817-3 (alk. paper)
 I. McKeon, Patrick O. (Patrick Owen), 1975- , editor. II. Wikstrom, Erik, A. (Erik Anders), 1978- , editor.
 [DNLM: 1. Ankle Injuries--therapy. 2. Sports Medicine--methods. WE 880]
 RD97
 617.1'027--dc23
                        2015000417

For permission to reprint material in another publication, contact SLACK Incorporated. Authorization to photocopy items for internal, personal, or academic use is granted by SLACK Incorporated provided that the appropriate fee is paid directly to the Copyright Clearance Center. Prior to photocopying items, please contact the Copyright Clearance Center at 222 Rosewood Drive, Danvers, MA 01923 USA; telephone: 978-750-8400; website: www.copyright.com; email: info@copyright.com

Printed in the United States of America.

Last digit is print number: 10   9   8   7   6   5   4   3   2   1

Quick Questions in
Ankle Sprains
Expert Advice in Sports Medicine

Quick Questions in Sports Medicine

Series

Series Editor, Eric L. Sauers, PhD, ATC, FNATA

Dedication

We would like to dedicate this book to our mentors, wives, children, parents, advisors, colleagues, and friends, who have helped us navigate life, love, and academia.

Contents

Section III Treatment and Rehabilitation 101

Acknowledgments

First and foremost, we must thank our contributors, whose international and multidisciplinary expertise has been at the forefront of caring for and advancing our knowledge regarding ankle joint pathologies. In addition, we must acknowledge the series editor, Eric Sauers, and thank him for the opportunity and his guidance while completing what we hope will be a tool to help clinicians improve their practice and patient outcomes. Finally, we must thank SLACK Incorporated and the individuals who do so much work behind the scenes.

About the Editors

Patrick O. McKeon, PhD, ATC, CSCS is an Assistant Professor in the Department of Exercise and Sport Sciences at Ithaca College and serves as the Clinical Education Coordinator for the Athletic Training Education program. Prior to coming to Ithaca College, Dr. McKeon served as an Assistant Professor within the Post-Professional Athletic Training program and the Rehabilitation Sciences Doctoral program at the University of Kentucky. He earned his bachelor of science degree in Athletic Training from Springfield College, his master of science in Sports Health Care from the Arizona School of Health Sciences, and his doctorate of philosophy in Sports Medicine from the University of Virginia. Dr. McKeon's research interests include understanding and enhancing recognition, prevention, and rehabilitation strategies for ankle instability. He incorporates a holistic research perspective, which combines patient-, clinician-, and laboratory-oriented outcomes to capture the broad spectrum of functional issues related to this clinical phenomenon.

Erik A. Wikstrom, PhD, ATC, FACSM is an Associate Professor in the Department of Kinesiology and the Co-Director of the Biodynamics Research Laboratory at UNC Charlotte. Prior to coming to UNC Charlotte, Dr. Wikstrom served as the Director of Undergraduate Athletic Training in the College of Health and Human Performance at the University of Florida. Dr. Wikstrom earned his bachelor of science degree in Athletic Training/Sports Medicine from Roanoke College and both his master of science degree in Exercise Science and his doctorate of philosophy in Health and Human Performance from the University of Florida. Dr. Wikstrom's research focuses on the interactions between musculoskeletal biomechanics and sensorimotor control of the lower extremity following injury, with particular emphasis on the coordination of balance in those with ankle joint pathologies.

Contributing Authors

Brent L. Arnold, PhD, ATC, FNATA
(Question 22)
Professor and Chair
Department of Health Sciences
Indiana University
School of Health and Rehabilitation
Sciences
Indianapolis, Indiana

Javier Beltran, MD (Question 18)
Chairman
Maimonides Medical Center
Department of Radiology
Brooklyn, New York

Chris M. Bleakley, PhD, BSc
(Questions 25, 31)
Physiotherapist and Lecturer
Ulster University
Faculty of Life and Health Science
Coleraine, United Kingdom

Cathleen N. Brown, PhD, ATC
(Question 13)
Associate Professor
University of Georgia
Kinesiology Department
College of Education
Athens, Georgia

Joshua Burns, PhD, BAppSc (Pod)(Hons)
(Questions 19, 33)
Professor of Paediatric Neuromuscular
Rehabilitation
Faculty of Health Sciences
The University of Sydney and The
Children's Hospital at Westmead
Sydney, Australia

Kenneth L. Cameron, PhD, MPH, ATC,
CSCS (Questions 4, 37)
Director of Orthopaedic Research
John A. Feagin Jr. Sports Medicine
Fellowship
Keller Army Hospital
United States Military Academy
West Point, New York

Brian Caulfield, PhD, M MedSc, B
Physio, MISCP (Question 16)
Professor of Physiotherapy
School of Public Health, Physiotherapy
and Population Science
University College Dublin
Dublin, Ireland

Lisa Chinn, PhD, AT (Question 5)
Assistant Professor of Athletic
Training
Department of Health Sciences
Kent State University
Kent, Ohio

*Mitchell L. Cordova, PhD, ATC,
   FNATA, FACSM (Question 7)*
Professor—Department of
   Rehabilitation Sciences
Dean—College of Health Professions
   and Social Work
Florida Gulf Coast University
Fort Myers, Florida

*Eamonn Delahunt, PhD, BSc
   (Physiotherapy), SMISCP
   (Question 16)*
Senior Lecturer
School of Public Health, Physiotherapy
   and Population Science
University College Dublin
Dublin, Ireland

*Carrie Docherty, PhD, ATC, FNATA
   (Question 17)*
Associate Professor
Department of Kinesiology
School of Public Health
Indiana University
Bloomington, Indiana

*Cailbhe Doherty, BSc (Physiotherapy)
   (Question 16)*
PhD Student
School of Public Health, Physiotherapy
   and Population Science
University College Dublin
Dublin, Ireland

*Michael G. Dolan, MA, ATC, CSCS
   (Question 21)*
Professor of Kinesiology
Canisius College
Department of Kinesiology
Buffalo, New York

Luke Donovan, PhD, ATC (Question 9)
Assistant Professor
University of Toledo
Department of Kinesiology
Toledo, Ohio

*Eric Eils, Prof. Dr. rer. medic. habil.
   (Question 28)*
Lecturer and Research Scientist
Institute of Sport and Exercise Sciences
Department of Psychology and Sport
   and Exercise Sciences
University of Muenster
Muenster, Germany

*J. Kent Ellington, MD, MS
   (Questions 36, 38)*
OrthoCarolina
Foot and Ankle Institute
Charlotte, North Carolina

Todd A. Evans, PhD, ATC (Question 34)
Associate Professor, Athletic Training
University of Northern Iowa
Human Performance Center
Cedar Falls, Iowa

Chad M. Ferguson, MD (Question 36)
Carolinas Medical Center
Department of Orthopaedic Surgery
Charlotte, North Carolina

*François Fourchet, PT, PhD
   (Question 27)*
Senior Physiotherapist
Hôpital La Tour Réseau de Soins
Meyrin/Geneva
Switzerland

Philip Glasgow, PhD, BSc (Question 25)
Director of Sports Medicine
Sports Institute of Northern Ireland
Ulster University
Coleraine, United Kingdom

Phillip Gribble, PhD, ATC, FNATA (Question 29)
Associate Professor
University of Kentucky
Division of Athletic Training
Department of Rehabilitation Sciences
Lexington, Kentucky

Jay Hertel, PhD, ATC (Question 9
Joe H. Gieck Professor of Sports Medicine
University of Virginia
Department of Kinesiology
Charlottesville, Virginia

Claire E. Hiller, PhD, MAppSc, BAppSc (Physio) (Questions 19, 33)
Research Fellow
Faculty of Health Sciences
The University of Sydney
Sydney, Australia

Matthew C. Hoch, PhD, ATC (Question 30)
Assistant Professor
School of Physical Therapy and Athletic Training
Old Dominion University
Norfolk, Virginia

J. Ty Hopkins, PhD, ATC, FNATA, FACSM (Question 15)
Professor
Exercise Sciences
Human Performance Research Center
Brigham Young University
Provo, Utah

Tricia Hubbard-Turner, PhD, ATC, FACSM (Question 20)
Associate Professor
Department of Kinesiology
University of North Carolina
Charlotte, North Carolina

Darren James, PhD (Question 27)
Lecturer in Biomechanics
School of Applied Sciences
London South Bank University
London, United Kingdom

Michael Johnson, PT, DSc, OCS, SCS (Question 37)
Assistant Director, US Military-Baylor University
Physical Therapy Sports Medicine Program
Keller Army Community Hospital
West Point, New York

Thomas W. Kaminski, PhD, ATC,
FNATA, FACSM (Question 11)
Editor—Athletic Training & Sports
  Health Care
Director of Athletic Training
  Education
Professor
University of Delaware
Department of Kinesiology and
  Applied Physiology
Newark, Delaware

Jupil Ko, MS, ATC (Question 13)
Doctoral Research Assistant
University of Georgia
Kinesiology Department
College of Education
Athens, Georgia

John E. Kovaleski, PhD, ATC
(Question 32)
Professor and Chair
Department of Health, Physical
  Education, & Leisure Studies
University of South Alabama
Mobile, Alabama

Tennyson Maliro, MD (Question 18)
Musculoskeletal Radiologist
vRad (Virtual Radiologic Professionals,
  LLC)
Eden Prairie, Minnesota

Carl G. Mattacola, PhD, ATC, FNATA
(Question 26)
Professor—Director Division of
  Athletic Training
Rehabilitation Sciences Doctoral
  Program
University of Kentucky
College of Health Sciences
Lexington, Kentucky

Timothy A. McGuine, PhD, ATC
(Question 6)
Senior Scientist
Division of Sports Medicine
Department of Orthopedics and
  Rehabilitation
University of Wisconsin School of
  Medicine and Public Health
Madison, Wisconsin

Jennifer M. Medina McKeon, PhD,
ATC, CSCS (Question 2)
Assistant Professor
Department of Exercise & Sport
  Sciences
School of Health Sciences & Human
  Performance
Ithaca College
Ithaca, New York

Eric Nussbaum, MEd, ATC, LAT
(Questions 11, 12)
Athletic Trainer
Freehold, New Jersey

Brett D. Owens, MD (Questions 4, 37)
LTC(P) MC USA
Professor, USUHS
John A. Feagin, Jr. Sports Medicine
   Fellowship
Keller Army Community Hospital
US Military Academy
West Point, New York

Kevin D. Phelps, MD (Question 38)
Resident Physician
Department of Orthopaedic Surgery
Carolinas Medical Center
Charlotte, North Carolina

Thomas L. Pommering, DO, FAAFP
   (Question 2)
Associate Clinical Professor of
   Pediatrics and Family Medicine
The Ohio State University College of
   Medicine
Division Chief for Sports Medicine
Nationwide Children's Hospital
Columbus, Ohio

Leah H. Portnow, MD (Question 18)
Radiology Resident
Maimonides Medical Center
Department of Radiology
Brooklyn, New York

Kelli Frye Pugh, MS, ATC, LMT
   (Question 35)
Associate Athletic Trainer
University of Virginia
Charlottesville, Virginia

Adam B. Rosen, PhD, ATC
   (Question 13)
Assistant Professor
University of Nebraska at Omaha
School of Health, Physical Education
   and Recreation
College of Education
Omaha, Nebraska

Scott E. Ross, PhD, LAT, ATC, FNATA
   (Question 22)
Associate Professor
Director, AT Program
University of North Carolina
   Greensboro
School of Health & Human Sciences
Department of Kinesiology
Greensboro, North Carolina

Helene Simpson, MSc Physiotherapy
   (Question 24)
Owner Physiotherapist
Sport Injuries Centre
University of Cape Town
Cape Town, South Africa

Kelli R. Snyder, EdD, ATC
   (Question 34)
Assistant Professor, Athletic Training
   Program Director
School of Health, Physical Education,
   and Leisure Services
Division of Athletic Training
University of Northern Iowa
Cedar Falls, Iowa

Matthew Stewart, PT, FACP
    (Question 10)
Specialist Sports Physiotherapist
Sports Physio West
Sydney, Australia

James C. Sullivan, DPM, ATC,
FACFAS (Question 12)
Foot and Ankle Consultant
Athletic Departments
University of Rhode Island
Providence College
Rhode Island College
Providence Bruins
United States Womans Gymnastics
North Smithfield, Rhode Island

Joseph Surace, DO (Question 18)
Musculoskeletal Radiologist
Schenectady Radiologists, PC
Schenectady, New York

Masafumi Terada, PhD, ATC
    (Question 29)
Postdoctoral Scholar
Department of Rehabilitation Science
College of Health Sciences
University of Kentucky
Lexington, Kentucky

Jeffrey D. Tiemstra, MD, FAAFP
    (Question 14)
Professor of Clinical Family Medicine
University of Illinois College of
    Medicine
Department of Family Medicine
University of Illinois Hospital and
    Health Sciences System
Chicago, Illinois

Evert Verhagen, PhD, FECSS
    (Question 8)
Associate Professor
VU University medical center
Department of Public and
    Occupational Health
Amsterdam, the Netherlands

Bill Vicenzino, PhD (Question 30)
Professor in Sports Physiotherapy
School of Health and Rehabilitation
    Sciences: Physiotherapy
The University of Queensland
Brisbane, Australia

Brian R. Waterman, MD (Question 4)
Director of Orthopaedic Research,
    Department of Orthopaedic Surgery
    and Rehabilitation, William
    Beaumont Army Medical Center, El
    Paso, Texas
Assistant Professor, Department of
    Orthopaedic Surgery, Texas Tech
    University Health Sciences Center,
    El Paso, Texas
Assistant Professor, Department
    of Surgery, Uniformed Services
    University of the Health Sciences,
    Bethesda, Maryland

Caitlin Whale, MS, LAT, ATC
    (Question 26)
Doctoral Student
University of Kentucky
College of Health Sciences
Department of Rehabilitation Sciences
Lexington, Kentucky

Tine Willems, PhD, PT (Question 3)
Post-Doctoral Scientific Researcher
Ghent University
Department of Orthopedics and
 Physiotherapy and Department of
 Rehabilitation Sciences and Physical
 Therapy
Ghent University Hospital
Ghent, Belgium

Matthew S. Wilson, MD (Question 39)
Resident Physician
Carolinas Medical Center
Department of Orthopaedic Surgery
Charlotte, North Carolina

Preface

The Quick Questions series was developed to provide clinicians with brief, direct, actionable answers to clinical questions that they encounter in the daily practice of sports medicine to help optimize patient care. Today, information access is easier than it has ever been. However, it is a challenge to find the time and develop the skill to consume and synthesize large bodies of evidence to distill knowledge into action. Because we typically do not have the time to complete this daunting task for every clinical question that arises, we often turn to our peers and colleagues for advice. One of the most trusted sources of information in health care is the expert consult. The Quick Questions series is like having a team of sports medicine experts with you on the sidelines or in the clinic to provide you with concise, straightforward advice to answer your most important clinical questions.

The editor of each book is a leading expert in his or her area of sports medicine practice who has assembled a team of expert clinicians and scholars to develop answers to 39 of the most commonly posed and clinically important questions. Each book is a compendium of expert advice from clinicians with the knowledge and experience to help guide your clinical decision making to provide safe and effective patient care.

In this book, *Quick Questions in Ankle Sprains: Expert Advice in Sports Medicine*, Drs. Patrick O. McKeon and Erik A. Wikstrom and their team of international expert contributing authors have answered 39 of the most important clinical questions for what is undoubtedly the most common injury encountered in the daily practice of athletic training and sports medicine. While the questions focus on lateral ankle sprains, appropriate attention is given to medial and syndesmotic sprains and the pediatric patient as well. This book begins with a series of important questions regarding the risk of lateral ankle sprains and key questions regarding risk reduction. Next, the focus turns to the diagnosis of ankle sprains, with a wealth of information including grading, diagnostic accuracy, functional testing, imaging, and the Ottawa Ankle and Foot Rules. The book then flows into a comprehensive series of questions regarding the treatment and rehabilitation of ankle sprains providing contemporary best practice recommendations to optimize patient outcomes and prevent recurrence. In addition to these foundational areas, this section provides expert advice on broader topics such as choosing patient-rated outcomes measures and treating cuboid syndrome. The final section of the book is dedicated to addressing important surgical considerations for treating ankle sprains.

With the busy schedules, job stresses, and time constraints inherent to sports medicine practice, it is my sincere hope that this series proves to be a valuable resource full of expert advice that you find helpful in caring for your patients and athletes.

Eric L. Sauers, PhD, ATC, FNATA
Series Editor

Introduction

The mission of the National Athletic Trainers' Association (NATA), which chartered the *Quick Question Series* in cooperation with SLACK Incorporated, is to enhance the quality of health care provided by certified athletic trainers and to advance the athletic training profession. Ankle sprains represent the most common orthopedic injury encountered by athletic trainers and therapists. At least 1 of every 3 people who suffer one ankle sprain continue to have functional problems including recurrent sprains, perceived instability, and decreased quality of life. The NATA, in conjunction with the International Ankle Consortium (IAC), has recognized the significant burden ankle sprains pose to those who seek to be physically active. We have developed and written this book in the spirit of the mission of the IAC, which is to advance the prevention, assessment, and treatment of ankle pathologies from a multidisciplinary perspective. The contributing authors of this book are all internationally recognized clinical researchers in their respective disciplines, and many of them are members of the IAC.

Quick Questions in Ankle Sprains is divided into 4 sections in which topics related to the prevention, assessment, rehabilitation, and surgical considerations for ankle sprains are concisely discussed. The authors of each of the questions were selected on the basis of their respective areas of expertise. The questions answered represent the most common questions posed by clinicians and patients who experience ankle sprains first hand. While each question is independent of the next, we encourage the reader to see the overlap in concepts, clinical trends, and research evidence as they relate to the 4 sections of this book. Because ankle sprains have such a high recurrence rate, we are constantly seeking to enhance our understanding in preventing and treating these injuries. We hope that new insights related to ankle sprain prevention, assessment, and treatment can be gleaned from the answers provided in this book.

SECTION I

RISK AND RISK REDUCTION OF ANKLE SPRAINS

WHY ARE LATERAL ANKLE SPRAINS SO COMMON IN SPORTS AND PHYSICAL ACTIVITY?

Erik A. Wikstrom, PhD, ATC, FACSM
and Patrick O. McKeon, PhD, ATC, CSCS

It is no secret that lateral ankle sprains are the most common musculoskeletal injury suffered during sports or physical activity regardless of age or activity. Indeed, an estimated half a million ankle sprains that warrant visits to the emergency department occur in the United States each year.[1] Amazingly, these injuries account for one third of the ankle sprains typically experienced. Some published data and certainly anecdotal evidence suggest that more than half of all individuals who sprain an ankle do not seek treatment from any health care professional[2]; thus, the true incidence of injury may be much greater.

But what is a lateral ankle sprain, and why is this injury so common? Lateral ankle sprains are also referred to as inversion ankle sprains or, occasionally, as supination ankle sprains. In the open kinetic chain, supination consists of plantar flexion, inversion, and internal rotation, while in the closed kinetic chain, supination consists of dorsiflexion, inversion, and internal rotation.[3] While the combined motions differ slightly, ankle sprains occur because of an inversion loading regardless of the sagittal plane position (dorsi flexion vs plantar flexion) of the ankle. Numerous individual factors could be argued regarding why ankle sprains are so common, but we will focus our response on 2 interconnecting concepts that are actually quite intuitive.

McKeon PO, Wikstrom EA, eds. *Quick Questions in Ankle Sprains: Expert Advice in Sports Medicine* (pp 3-6).
© 2015 SLACK Incorporated.

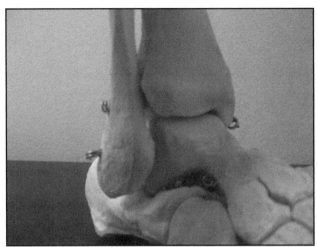

Figure 1-1. The ankle in a closed packed position providing good congruity of the articular surfaces and restraint against excessive talar motion.

The first concept is the most well known to health care providers and deals directly with ankle anatomy. More specifically, the insufficiencies of the major contributors toward ankle joint stability: (1) the congruity of the bony surfaces when the joint is loaded, (2) the static stabilizers (ligaments), and (3) the dynamic stabilizers (muscles).[3] When the ankle is in a loaded and closed packed position (ie, dorsiflexed), the articular surfaces are the primary restraint against excessive talar rotation and translation. In this position, the ankle is very stable, assuming there is no frontal plane movement. However, the congruence of the talar dome relative to the distal articulating surfaces of the tibia and fibula (the mortise) decreases as the foot is plantar flexed, resulting in less bony stabilization (Figures 1-1 and 1-2). However, when the ankle plantar flexes, the joint is still well protected against medial ankle sprains because of the length of the lateral malleolus (ie, its projection inferiorly beyond the ankle joint), which provides a bony block against eversion. The relatively short medial malleolus fails to provide such a bony block against inversion motion, which further increases the likelihood of a lateral ankle sprain, especially when the ankle is plantar flexed. Thus, during physical activity of any kind, which always requires some degree of plantar flexion, the ankle is forced to rely on the static and dynamic stabilizers rather than on the bony congruency of the talus and mortise to prevent lateral ankle sprains.

Based on the bony anatomy, the static stabilizers are crucial for providing joint stability. The lateral static stabilizers include the joint capsule, the anterior talofibular ligament (ATFL), the posterior talofibular ligament, and the calcaneofibular ligament (CFL). Research has shown that the ATFL prevents anterior displacement of the talus from the mortise and excessive inversion and internal rotation

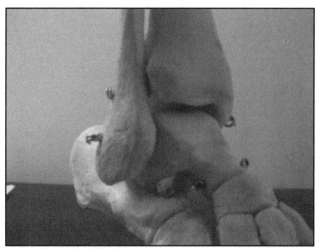

Figure 1-2. The ankle in a plantar flexed and open packed position demonstrating the decreased congruence of the articular surfaces.

of the talus on the tibia.[3] Unfortunately, the ATFL is the weakest of the lateral ligaments and suffers the greatest strain as the ankle moves into plantar flexion. This is an important shortcoming of the static stabilizers. Because of the strain already placed on the ATFL when the foot is plantar flexed, it is not capable of absorbing the additional forces placed upon it when an inversion loading (ie, sprain mechanism) begins to occur, which is one possible reason why the ATFL is the most frequently injured of the lateral ligaments. The CFL restricts excessive inversion and internal rotation, but it is most taut when the ankle is dorsiflexed. Thus, if bony congruence fails when dorsiflexed, the CFL is already stressed and limited in its ability to absorb the additional forces placed upon it during an inversion loading mechanism.

Finally, the dynamic stabilizers generate stiffness during activity to protect the joints. The primary stabilizers are the peroneal longus and brevis muscles, the primary role of which is to evert the foot or to control supination eccentrically while weight bearing. However, there is a controversy about whether the peroneal muscles are actually able to respond quickly enough to prevent an ankle sprain.[4] The peroneals may not respond the same way when performing a very controlled movement in a laboratory compared to dynamic tasks during real-life situations. Regardless of the speed at which the peroneals react, the amount of force that they can handle is a separate but equally important factor. In addition to the peroneals, the anterior tibialis, extensor digitorum longus, extensor digitorum brevis, and peroneus tertius are also believed to assist in providing dynamic stability of the lateral ankle complex by slowing the plantar-flexion component of supination, but we are less than certain that this function occurs during dynamic motions. In summary, the 3 major sources of ankle joint stability have limitations that unfortunately often occur simultaneously and especially when coupled with the remaining concepts and create opportunities for lateral ankle sprains during physical activity and sport.

The second concept deals with the fact that the foot-ankle complex is the singular point of contact between the body and support surface during every step taken during physical activity and sporting events. Thus, the sheer number of steps taken during physical activity (eg, > 2000 steps to walk 1 mile) increases the opportunity for the lateral ligaments of the ankle to be sprained. Such a sprain may be the result of an internal perturbation (eg, an incorrectly timed muscle contraction), an external perturbation (eg, stepping in a hole or on a foot), or the interactions between them.

So why are lateral ankle sprains so common? Quite simply, the foot-ankle complex is subjected to high-impact multidirectional forces during physical activity and sport when in positions that highlight specific anatomical shortcomings. The result is a high volume of lateral ankle sprains as evidenced by epidemiological data. Unfortunately, lateral ankle sprains have a very high recurrence rate, and many individuals who suffer a lateral ankle sprain (~30% to 40%) develop chronic ankle instability (CAI).[5] Also, CAI has been linked to the development of posttraumatic ankle osteoarthritis. Given the frequency of lateral ankle sprains and potential for long-term consequences, proper diagnosis and treatment of acute lateral ankle sprains, CAI, and concomitant injuries are of primary importance.

References

1. Waterman BR, Owens BD, Davey S, Zacchilli MA, Belmont PJ, Jr. The epidemiology of ankle sprains in the United States. *J Bone Joint Surg Am.* 2010;92:2279-2284.
2. McKay GD. Ankle injuries in basketball: injury rate and risk factors. *Br J Sports Med.* 2001;35:103-108.
3. Hertel J. Functional anatomy, pathomechanics, and pathophysiology of lateral ankle instability. *J Athl Train.* 2002;37:364-375.
4. Hoch MC, McKeon PO. Peroneal reaction time and ankle sprain risk in healthy adults: a critically appraised topic. *J Sport Rehab.* 2011;20:505-511.
5. Wikstrom EA, Hubbard-Turner T, McKeon PO. Understanding and treating lateral ankle sprains and their consequences: a constraints-based approach. *Sports Med.* 2013;43:385-393.

HOW DOES THE INCIDENCE OF LATERAL ANKLE SPRAINS DIFFER ACROSS SPORTS AND PHYSICAL ACTIVITIES?

Jennifer M. Medina McKeon, PhD, ATC, CSCS
and Thomas L. Pommering, DO, FAAFP

The goal of this chapter is inform the clinician about when and how ankle sprains are most likely to happen. Ankle sprains are the most common injury in sports; this has been demonstrated repeatedly. From this evidence alone, the clinician can generate a list of differential diagnoses when there is an injury at the foot-ankle complex, and an ankle sprain should be included in the differential diagnosis. But beyond that, an epidemiological approach can be used to determine what sports a clinician should expect to see an even greater number of ankle sprains. To illustrate this, the literature has been summarized in regards to the most popular sports (by participation numbers) and by the expectation of ankle sprains within those sports.

As the tables are inspected, the readers should pay close attention to a couple of meaningful points:

- The *ranking* provides the information as to the most at-risk sports for ankle sprain.

- The *injury rate* details the magnitude of the injury problem and allows the clinician to contrast their own ankle sprain injury rates compared to national data.

McKeon PO, Wikstrom EA, eds. *Quick Questions in
Ankle Sprains: Expert Advice in Sports Medicine* (pp 7-14).
© 2015 SLACK Incorporated.

- The *percentage of all injuries* offers information about the size of the ankle sprain problem compared to other injuries.

Adult Population

Ankle sprains are the most common sports-related injury. For adults and adolescents, males and females, ankle sprains are frequent and therefore, should be anticipated when evaluating an injury to the lower extremity. That being said, the problem of ankle sprain can be further evaluated within specific populations and sports. In particular, sports that require sprinting, quick changes in direction, and jumping are those for which ankle sprains are most prevalent. Sports such as football, basketball, soccer, and volleyball—those which require these types of movements—are the sports which have the highest incidence of ankle sprain. Based on the inherent nature of these sports and the body types of the athletes who tend to participate in them, there are many nonmodifiable risk factors that increase the chances of ankle sprain. However, there are also modifiable risk factors for ankle sprains that should be considered and addressed by the practicing clinician, when appropriate. Being able to predict which sports have the highest incidence of ankle sprains is helpful to athletic trainers, team physicians, and event organizers who are planning and providing medical care for these athletes.

Tables 2-1 and 2-2 represent the sports-related ankle sprain problem for both male and female adult athletes (National Collegiate Athletic Association [NCAA] and international data). For adult males, at both the NCAA and at international levels, the same 4 sports (football, soccer, basketball, lacrosse) appear as sports that place the athlete at a higher risk for ankle sprains. For women, at both the NCAA and international levels, the same 4 sports (soccer, basketball, volleyball, lacrosse) appear as sports that place the athlete at risk for ankle sprains.

RANKING

Interestingly, 5 sports overall (football, soccer, basketball, volleyball, and lacrosse) have the highest incidence of ankle sprains for both men and women. These are also some of the most popular sports in the world. Not surprisingly, these sports also incorporate the same types of movements and styles of play; sprinting, jumping, and cutting are inherent to participation in these sports.

INJURY RATE

Ankle sprain injury rates have been reported for the NCAA, and for the 5 sports with the highest numbers of ankle sprains, the injury rates range from around 0.70 to 1.30 injuries per 1000 athlete-exposures. In other words, if a clinician

Table 2-1				
Top 10 Men's Sports (by Participation Numbers) and Ankle Sprain Epidemiology				
	NCAA		International	
Top Men's Sports (Based on Participation Numbers)[3]	*Ankle Sprain Injury Rank and Rate (per 1000 Athlete-Exposures [95% CIs])[4]*	*Ankle Sprain Injury Rank as Percentage of All Injuries[4]*	*Ankle Sprain Injury Rank as Percentage of All Injuries[5]*	*Ankle Sprain Injury Rank as a Percentage of All Ankle Injuries[5]*
1 **Football**	#3: 0.83[.81,.84]	#4: 13.6	#3: 16.0%	**#1: 94.4%**
2 Track and field			5.5%	48.9%
3 Baseball				
4 **Soccer**	#2: 1.24[1.19,1.29]	#2: 17.2	#1: 16.3%	**#4: 76.8%**
5 **Basketball**	#1: 1.30[1.26,1.35]	#1: 26.6	#4: 14.5%	**#2: 91.0%**
6 Cross country			5.5%	48.9%
7 **Lacrosse**	#4: 0.66[0.61,0.71]	#3: 14.4	#2: 16.2%	**#3: 87.5%**
8 Swimming and diving				
9 Golf				
10 Tennis			5.3%	66.7%

has 100 athletes participating every day for 10 days, this would be equivalent to 1000 athlete-exposures. That clinician should expect around one ankle sprain during that time.

PERCENTAGE OF ALL INJURIES

As a percentage of all injuries, ankle sprains are all too common—for the top 5 sports with the highest number of sprains, the percentage of ankle sprains is 14% of all injuries or higher. For women's volleyball, ankle sprains account for almost half of all injuries. To summarize, ankle sprains occur in substantial numbers, accounting for large percentages of all injuries that occur in sports.

Table 2-2

Top 10 Women's Sports (by Participation Numbers) and Ankle Sprain Epidemiology

		NCCA		International	
	Top Women's Sports (Based on Participation Numbers)[3]	Ankle Sprain Injury Rank and Rate (per 1000 Athlete-Exposures [95% CIs])[4]	Ankle Sprain Injury Rank as Percentage of all Injuries[4]	Ankle Sprain Injury Rank as Percentage of all Injuries[5]	Ankle Sprain Injury Rank as a Percentage of all Ankle Injuries[5]
1	Track and field			5.5%	48.9%
2	**Soccer**	#1: 1.30[1.24,1.36]	#4: 16.7	#2: 16.3%	**#4: 76.8%**
3	Softball				
4	**Basketball**	#2: 1.15[1.10,1.20]	#1: 24.0	#4: 14.5%	**#2: (91.0%**
5	**Volleyball**	#3: 1.01[0.96,1.06]	#2: 23.8	#1: 45.3%	**#1: (99.3%**
6	Cross country			5.5%	48.9%
7	Swimming and diving				
8	Tennis			5.3%	66.7%
9	**Lacrosse**	#4: 0.70[0.65,0.76]	#3: 17.7	#3: 16.2%	**#3: 87.5%**
10	Rowing				

Adolescent Population

At the high school level, ankle sprains are also a considerable problem; approximately 20%[1,2] of all injures (17.5% for boys and 25% for girls)[1] are ankle sprains.

For high school sports, ankle sprain injury data have reported in varied fashions in the literature. This information has been summarized and ankle sprain injury problem is presented below, again, for the top 10 sports for boys and girls based on participation numbers (Tables 2-3 and 2-4). Although ankle sprains as a percentage of all injuries was not reported, an estimate of these percentages has been calculated. Using the published ankle sprain injury rates (per 10,000 athlete-exposures) and published all sports-related injury rates (per 10,000 athlete-exposures), estimate percentages have been calculated.

Table 2-3

Top 10 Boys' Sports (by Participation Numbers) and Ankle Sprain Epidemiology

		Estimated Percentage = Ankle Sprain Injury Rate ÷ All Sports-Related Injuries Injury Rate		
	Top Boys' High School Sports (Based on Participation Numbers)	*Ankle Sprain Injury Rank and Rate (per 10,000 Athlete-Exposures)[2]*	*All Sports-Related Injuries Injury Rate (per 10,000 AE)[6]*	*Estimated Percentage of Ankle Sprains*
1	**Football**	#2: 4.7	43.6	10.8%
2	Track and field	0.5	N/R	Not calculated
3	**Basketball**	#1: 5.2	18.9	27.5%
4	Baseball	0.9	11.9	7.6%
5	**Soccer**	#3: 3.1	24.3	12.8%
6	Wrestling	#4: 1.4	25.0	5.6%
7	Cross country	N/R	N/R	Not calculated
8	Tennis	N/R	N/R	Not calculated
9	Golf	N/R	N/R	Not calculated
10	Swimming and diving	0.00	N/R	Not calculated

RANKING

Compared to adult males, high school age males have the same top 3 sports for risk of ankle sprain (basketball, football, and soccer). Likewise, compared to adult females, high school age females have the same top 3 sports for risk of ankle sprain (soccer, basketball, and volleyball).

INJURY RATE

While the ranking of the most at-risk sports are comparable between adults and adolescent, there was a substantial decrease in the ankle sprain injury rates for adolescents. Based on the injury rates for the top 3 sports at the high school level, clinicians should expect 3 to 5 ankle sprains per 10,000 athlete-exposures.

		Estimated Percentage = Ankle Sprain Injury Rate ÷ All Sports-Related Injuries Injury Rate		
	Top Girls' High School Sports (Based on Participation Numbers)	**Ankle Sprain Injury Rank and Rate (per 10,000 Athlete-Exposures)[2]**	**All Sports-Related Injuries Injury Rate (per 10,000 AE)[6]**	**Estimated Percentage of Ankle Sprains**
1	Track and Field	0.98	N/R	Not calculated
2	**Basketball**	#1: 5.03	20.1	25.0%
3	**Volleyball**	#3: 3.90	16.4	23.8%
4	**Soccer**	#2: 4.59	23.6	19.3%
5	Softball	1.50	11.3	12.3%
6	Cross Country	N/R	N/R	Not calculated
7	Tennis	N/R	N/R	Not calculated
8	Swimming and Diving	0.06	N/R	Not calculated
9	Cheerleading	0.68	N/R	Not calculated
10	Lacrosse	#4: 2.45	N/R	Not calculated

Table 2-4

Top 10 Girls' Sports (by Participation Numbers) and Ankle Sprain Epidemiology

PERCENTAGE OF ALL INJURIES

As a percentage of all injuries, ankle sprains represent a considerable proportion of injuries. For boys' sports, clinicians should expect around 15% of all injuries to be ankle sprains. For girls' sports, this number reaches an estimate of 25%.

Summary of Adolescent and Adult Population

It is interesting and important to note that at both the adolescent and adult competition levels, we can expect a similar pattern of at-risk sports for ankle sprain. Even though the progression of levels of competition from high school to more advanced play, the frequency of ankle sprains appears to be consistent in selected sports. Based on the evidence, it appears that there are inherent factors within these sports that contribute to an increased injury risk compared to other sports regardless of their age or ability level.

Sport-Specific Contributing Factors for Ankle Sprains

Across all of the populations examined here (males and females, adult and adolescent), there were similarities among the sports that are most risk for ankle sprains (football, soccer, basketball, volleyball, and lacrosse). Certainly, there are several modifiable and nonmodifiable risk factors that may explain the high prevalence of ankle sprains within these sports. More specifically, there are nonmodifiable *sport* and *athlete* factors to consider. Nonmodifiable sport factors include the physical demands and inherent conditions under which the sport is played. Sports that require play in close proximity to other players in which direct contact with another player's foot is likely, jumping and landing are common, or quick directional changes are necessary are all inherent within these sports. Nonmodifiable athlete risk factors, such as being taller and heavier, have been demonstrated to increase the risk for ankle sprains. Unquestionably, taller and heavier athletes tend to be seen in basketball, football, and volleyball—those sports with high risk of ankle sprain—when compared to sports with lower ankle sprain incidence. It is worth noting that, anatomically, the posterior aspect of the talus is narrower than the anterior. As such, when athletes are landing from a jump they are initially in plantar flexion and positioned over the narrower posterior talus where the surface area is smaller, making inversion or eversion more likely to occur if other factors such as contact with another player or stepping on another player's foot is possible.

Finally, some modifiable risk factors include aspects such as the type and/or condition of playing surface, weather conditions that could affect outdoor venues, and exposure to foul play. Uneven playing surfaces, especially those affected by changing conditions throughout the contest, as seen in football, soccer and lacrosse, would make the risk for ankle sprains increase. Additionally, with the exception of volleyball, sports with the highest incidence of ankle sprains are contact or collision sports where emotions and foul play may play a role. While both modifiable and nonmodifiable factors play a role in increasing the potential risk for ankle sprains, it is important to consider which factors can be changed. Further discussion on the risk factors for ankle sprains and the ability to modify them are further discussed in Questions 3 and 4.

References

1. Fernandez WG, Yard EE, Comstock RD. Epidemiology of lower extremity injuries among US high school athletes. *Acad Emerg Med.* 2007;14:641-645.
2. Swenson DM, Collins CL, Fields SK, Comstock RD. Epidemiology of US high school sports-related ligamentous ankle injuries, 2005/06–2010/11. *Clin J Sports Med.* 2013;23:190-196.
3. National Collegiate Athletic Association. *1981-82 - 2010-11 NCAA Sports Sponsorship and Participation Rates Report.* Indianapolis, IN: National Collegiate Athletic Association; 2008.
4. Hootman J, Dick R, Agel J. Epidemiology of collegiate injuries for 15 sports: summary and recommendations for injury prevention initiatives. *J Athl Train.* 2007;42:311-319.
5. Fong DT, Hong Y, Chan LK, Yung PS, Chan KM. A systematic review on ankle injury and ankle sprain in sports. *Sports Med.* 2007;37:73-94.
6. Centers for Disease Control and Prevention. Sports-related injuries among high school athletes-United States 2005-06 school year. *MMWR Morb Mortal Wkly Rep.* 2006;55:1037-1040.

WHAT ARE THE MOST COMMON MODIFIABLE RISK FACTORS FOR LATERAL ANKLE SPRAINS?

Tine Willems, PhD, PT

Lateral ankle sprains are very common injuries that can lead to physical and emotional impairments in the short term and have a high potential to progress to permanent disability in the long term. Nearly half of the sprains occur during athletic activity, and the peak incidence of ankle sprains is among adolescents and young adults. Many ankle sprains are a result of unavoidable accidents, but there are also many others that could be prevented. Because ankle sprains are so prevalent in sports, it is important to identify risk factors to ultimately prevent these injuries.

Any factor increasing the chance of an injury is considered a risk factor. Risk factors for ankle sprains are multifactorial and are traditionally divided into 1 of 2 main categories: intrinsic and extrinsic risk factors. The intrinsic risk factors are related to individual biological or psychosocial characteristics such as age, joint stability, muscle strength, muscle tightness, biomechanics, conditioning, previous injuries, adequacy of rehabilitation, and psychosocial stress. Extrinsic risk factors relate to environmental variables such as level of play, exercise load (type, intensity, and amount of physical activity), position played, and equipment used. Both intrinsic and extrinsic risk factors can partially influence each other and are therefore not independent of each other. Most of the time, a collection of risk factors interact and produce sufficient cause for an injury to occur.

McKeon PO, Wikstrom EA, eds. *Quick Questions in Ankle Sprains: Expert Advice in Sports Medicine* (pp 15-18). © 2015 SLACK Incorporated.

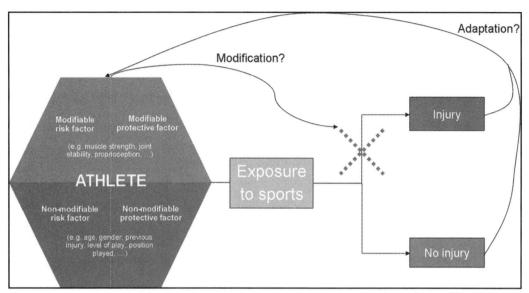

Figure 3-1. A new model of etiology in sport injury representing the relationship between modifiable and nonmodifiable risk and protective factors.

Sports injury researchers have traditionally conceptualized risk factors as intrinsic or extrinsic. Although intrinsic and extrinsic risk factors are important to address, it seems more important to understand those factors that can and cannot be changed. Therefore, a more favorable way of conceptualizing risk factors as modifiable or nonmodifiable has been used recently.[1] Although nonmodifiable risk factors such as gender and age may be of interest, it is important to study factors that are potentially modifiable through physical training or behavioral approaches.

Besides risk factors, an athlete also possesses protective factors that decrease the chance of an injury. A new conceptual model representing these risk and protective factors is introduced in Figure 3-1.

In practice, each athlete has his or her own particular set of risk and protective factors. It is the presence of both modifiable and nonmodifiable risk factors as well as their interaction that renders the athlete susceptible to injury, but the mere presence of these factors is usually not sufficient to produce injury. On the other hand, both modifiable and nonmodifiable protective factors may even prevent the occurrence of an injury. Additionally, one exposure to a potential inciting event can also alter an athlete's modifiable and nonmodifiable factors and change his or her predisposition to injury. Most important, however, is to prevent injuries from occurring. Adaptation of the modifiable risk factors into protective factors seems to be the best approach and should be the goal in injury prevention. Although clinically relevant, not much research has been done on protective risk factors for ankle sprains, and further research into protective risk factors is therefore warranted.

Identifying risk factors is not easy. The best way to determine risk factors is the prospective study design in which potential risk factors are measured before injuries occur, after which cases are reported during a period of follow-up. However, the main disadvantage of this study design is that study size is critical, because it is necessary to include and monitor a large number of subjects for an exceedingly long study period. This is the main reason why there are few prospective studies in the literature focusing on identifying risk factors for ankle sprains.

A recent meta-analysis[2] reviewed prospective studies investigating intrinsic functional deficits associated with increased risk of ankle injuries. Strength deficits in the lower leg musculature were revealed to be significant, but with relatively small effect sizes. Both decreased eccentric inversion strength and increased concentric plantar flexion increased the risk for an ankle sprain. In addition, the postural control variables were also significant, with a larger effect size. There was evidence to support a 2-fold increase in the risk based on a balance deficit. Another determined risk factor with a small effect size was decreased proprioception. Relatively poor active position–replication joint position sense performance in inversion was associated with an increased risk for ankle injury. In most studies, an increased body mass and increased weight were not identified as risk factors; however, in football players, these parameters did increase the risk for an ankle sprain. On the other hand, in recruits who have to carry heavy loads, a low body mass has been identified as a risk factor for ankle sprains. Muscle reaction time has also been studied a couple of times, but no clear association could be established. Next to this, range of ankle motions to plantar flexion, dorsiflexion, inversion and eversion, and ligament stability did not show a link to ankle injury risk.

In basketball players, inadequate warm-up has been identified as a risk factor for ankle injury.

Only a few studies have investigated biomechanical risk factors. These studies in Royal Marine recruits and physical education students identified a more medially directed pressure distribution during the stance phase in running as a risk factor.

Table 3-1 summarizes the modifiable risk factors for ankle sprains and possible recommendations for adaptation.

One of the most important and well-established risk factors for ankle sprains is a history of an ankle sprain. History is a nonmodifiable risk factor that is discussed in Question 4. However, because prevention of a first-time injury to an ankle will also prevent subsequent reinjury, this needs special attention.

Each of the previously performed studies on risk factors for ankle sprains had multiple inherent limitations and is likely to provide incomplete answers about complex, multifactorial injury conditions. Specifically, modifiable factors may change over time, and it is important to highlight that there is no clear evidence that any one particular risk factor is greater than another, and they are not

Table 3-1

Modifiable Risk Factors for Ankle Sprains and Possible Recommendations

Modifiable Risk Factor	Possible Recommendation for Adaptation
Decreased lower leg muscle strength	Strengthening exercises
Decreased postural control	Balance training
Decreased proprioception	Proprioceptive training
Medially directed pressure distribution during running	Adequate shoes or orthoses
Inadequate warm-up	Adequate warm-up

structurally linked with each other. However, on the basis of the evidence, screening for strength, balance, and proprioceptive deficits, assessing the roll-off pattern during running, and evaluating the preparation of an athlete/recruit prior to engaging in physical activity appear to be the most appropriate assessments of risk.

In the literature, the methods used to measure these risk factors are selected according to their reliability and validity. However, most of these methods use expensive equipment such as isokinetic dynamometers, balance platforms, and three-dimensional gait analysis systems. Until now, no research has been done to identify more user-friendly and less expensive tools to evaluate these risk factors in clinical practice. This makes it difficult at the moment to make recommendations for evaluating these risk factors in the clinical setting.

Establishing risk factors is one step. More important is the identification of high-risk subjects and modification of risk factors by introducing preventive measures. The role of sports medicine clinicians, athletic trainers, and strength and conditioning specialists should be to measure and train specific deficits in subjects susceptible to ankle sprains. Special attention should be given to decreased lower leg muscle strength, balance deficits, and decreased proprioception. Also, a proper warm-up and adequate shoes are helpful.

References

1. Cameron KL. Time for a paradigm shift in conceptualizing risk factors in sports injury research. *J Athl Train.* 2010;45:58-60.
2. Witchalls J, Blanch P, Waddington G, Adams R. Intrinsic functional deficits associated with increased risk of ankle injuries: a systematic review with meta-analysis. *Br J Sports Med.* 2012;46:515-523.

WHAT ARE THE MOST COMMON NONMODIFIABLE RISK FACTORS FOR LATERAL ANKLE SPRAINS?

Kenneth L. Cameron, PhD, MPH, ATC, CSCS;
Brian R. Waterman, MD; and Brett D. Owens, MD

Lateral ankle sprain injuries are one of the most common injuries experienced in sport, and they can often result in significant time lost to injury and long-term morbidity. While the modifiable risk factors for lateral ankle sprains serve as important targets for injury-prevention interventions, nonmodifiable risk factors are equally important for identifying individuals and populations who are at the greatest risk for injury.[1] In addition to establishing those who are most likely to sustain lateral ankle sprains, this information can also serve to inform screening guidelines and preventative measures, particularly in the presence of other modifiable risk factors (eg, poor balance or neuromuscular control). The purpose of this chapter is to provide an overview of the most common nonmodifiable risk factors for lateral ankle sprains, which include sex, age, injury history, generalized joint hypermobility, foot and ankle anatomy, and activity type. Clinically, this information should aid in identifying individuals and populations who are at the greatest risk for injury and those who should benefit most from injury screening and injury-prevention initiatives.

McKeon PO, Wikstrom EA, eds. *Quick Questions in Ankle Sprains: Expert Advice in Sports Medicine* (pp 19-23).
© 2015 SLACK Incorporated.

Sex

Females may be at greater risk for ankle sprain injuries than males. Prospective epidemiological studies suggest that incidence rates and prevalence estimates for ankle sprains among females are significantly higher than those among males.[2] Specifically, females appear to be twice as likely to experience an ankle sprain than males. However, many studies that have compared males and females have not specifically compared the incidence rates of ankle sprain among males and females in gender-matched sports (eg, soccer, basketball) with similar rules and physical activity requirements. This is important, because activity-related risk factors may not be the same when comparing males and females across different sports. Regardless, on the basis of what we currently know, clinicians should consider focusing screening and prevention efforts on young female athletes, particularly those engaged in high-risk activities.

Age

Age is also an important nonmodifiable risk factor associated with the incidence of lateral ankle sprain injuries.[2,3] Children experience the highest incidence rates for ankle sprain, followed by adolescents and adults, respectively.[2] The incidence rate for ankle sprains among children is 47% higher than the rate among adolescents and 10.5 times as high as the rate among adults.[2] While the incidence rate of ankle sprains is lower among adolescents than children, adolescents are still 7 times more likely to sustain an ankle sprain than adults.[2] A large epidemiological study examining the incidence rate of ankle sprains among active-duty military personnel also suggests that incidence rates are the highest in those less than 20 years of age, irrespective of gender, and rates generally decrease with increasing age.[3] Younger age groups, particularly those with other modifiable (eg, poor balance) and nonmodifiable (eg, high-risk activity such as basketball or soccer) risk factors for lateral ankle sprains, should be targeted for injury screening and primary prevention efforts. This is especially important considering the effect that injury history has on the risk for future ankle sprain, as noted in the next section.

Injury History

Athletes with a history of injury are much more likely to experience a second ankle sprain than those with no prior history of injury.[4] However, it remains unclear if the increased risk following an initial injury is due to preinjury factors, tissue damage at the time of injury, inadequate rehabilitation outcomes, or an interaction among these factors. Regardless, primary prevention efforts are critical in mitigating the morbidity and long-term consequences associated with lateral ankle sprain injuries in high-risk populations. Furthermore, athletes with a history of ankle sprain should be targeted for secondary prevention interventions such as prophylactic bracing and exercises to improve proprioception, postural control, strength, and mobility at the ankle joint.

Generalized Joint Hypermobility

Although there are some conflicting results, well-designed prospective studies suggest that generalized joint hypermobility is an important nonmodifiable risk factor for lateral ankle sprains.[5] Generalized joint hypermobility is usually assessed using the Beighton-Horan criteria for generalized joint hypermobility, and acute ankle sprains and chronic ankle instability are common in athletes with generalized joint hypermobility. Excessive ankle joint laxity has been reported in up to 93% of individuals in this population. Furthermore, the cumulative incidence of lateral ankle sprains has been reported to be over twice as high in athletes with generalized joint hypermobility than in their nonhypermobile counterparts.[5] Increased medial forefoot collapse during gait has also been observed in soccer players with generalized joint hypermobility, which is believed to contribute to ankle instability and a higher incidence of ankle sprain, as well as muscular problems due to the decreased mechanical advantage of the peroneous longus.[5] Athletes with generalized joint hypermobility, as assessed by the Beighton-Horan criteria, should be targeted for injury-prevention interventions that focus on strengthening the secondary stabilizers of the ankle joint and improving balance and proprioception.

Foot and Ankle Anatomy

Lower-extremity malalignment, particularly of the hindfoot or ankle, may predispose individuals to lateral ankle sprain injuries.[6] With reduced hindfoot mobility, varus malalignment, or a rigid cavus foot, the normal loading mechanics during gait are altered, leading to increased adduction and inversion forces about the ankle. Similarly, tarsal coalitions that restrict normal subtalar joint motion may predispose adolescent patients to lateral ankle sprains. Some evidence suggests that a posteriorly positioned fibula or fixed limitations in ankle dorsiflexion are additional nonmodifiable anatomic risk factors associated with lateral ankle sprains. While some of these morphological abnormalities about the ankle mortise may be difficult to screen for clinically, individuals with these conditions may benefit from preventive interventions.

Activity Type

Some may argue that activity type is a modifiable risk factor, particularly when initially deciding whether to participate in a specific sport; however, most experienced athletes would not choose to give up their sport because of an increased risk of lateral ankle sprain. As a result, we have elected to treat activity type as a nonmodifiable risk factor for lateral ankle sprain. The evidence clearly indicates that athletes who participate in sports and physical activities that require running, cutting, jumping, or quick and unanticipated changes in direction are at increased risk for lateral ankle sprain.[2,7] A recent meta-analysis of prospective epidemiological studies suggests that athletes who participate in indoor and court sports (eg, basketball or tennis) experience the highest incidence rates for lateral ankle sprain, followed by ice/water sports (eg, ice hockey or skiing), field sports (eg, football or field hockey), and other outdoor sports (eg, orienteering or track and field).[2] Ensuring that facilities are free of hazards, including debris on courts, and pot holes or uneven surfaces on playing fields used in high-risk activities can mitigate the risks in these sports. Athletes participating in high-risk activities should be targeted for injury screening and primary injury-prevention interventions including exercises to improve neuromuscular control and balance and prophylactic ankle bracing or taping.

Conclusion

Nonmodifiable risk factors for lateral ankle sprains are important for identifying individuals and populations who are at the greatest risk for injury so that they can be targeted for injury screening and prevention interventions. The most common nonmodifiable risk factors for lateral ankle sprains include female sex, younger age, a history of previous ankle sprain, generalized joint hypermobility, lower-extremity morphological abnormalities, and participation in sports and physical activities that require running, cutting, jumping, and quick and unanticipated changes in direction. We recommend that clinicians pay particular attention to athletes who fit this profile in clinical practice. For example, young females with generalized joint hypermobility and a history of previous ankle sprain and who are participating in soccer or basketball should be identified through preparticipation screening and targeted for appropriate injury-prevention interventions (eg, prophylactic bracing or taping and exercises to strengthen the secondary stabilizers of the ankle joint and improve balance and proprioception).

References

1. Cameron KL. Time for a paradigm shift in conceptualizing risk factors in sports injury research. *J Athl Train*. 2010;45:58-60.
2. Doherty C, Delahunt E, Caulfield B, et al. The incidence and prevalence of ankle sprain injury: a systematic review and meta-analysis of prospective epidemiological studies. *Sports Med*. 2014;44:123-140.
3. Cameron KL, Owens BD, DeBerardino TM. Incidence of ankle sprains among active-duty members of the United States Armed Services from 1998 through 2006. *J Athl Train*. 2010;45:29-38.
4. Kucera KL, Marshall SW, Kirkendall DT, Marchak PM, Garrett WE Jr. Injury history as a risk factor for incident injury in youth soccer. *Br J Sports Med*. 2005;39:462.
5. Wolf JM, Cameron KL, Owens BD. Impact of joint laxity and hypermobility on the musculoskeletal system. *J Am Acad Orthop Surg*. 2011;19:463-471.
6. Waterman BR, Langston JR, Cameron KL, Belmont PJ Jr, Owens BD. Sprain in the forecast: epidemiology and risk factors for ankle sprain. *Low Extrem Rev*. 2011:April;5-10.
7. Waterman BR, Belmont PJ, Jr, Cameron KL, Deberardino TM, Owens BD. Epidemiology of ankle sprain at the United States Military Academy. *Am J Sports Med*. 2010;38(4):797-803.

WHAT ARE THE CONTRIBUTING FACTORS FOR RECURRENT ANKLE SPRAINS AND/OR CHRONIC ANKLE INSTABILITY?

Lisa Chinn, PhD, AT

Chronic ankle instability (CAI) is most traditionally defined as repetitive bouts of lateral ankle instability resulting in numerous ankle sprains.[1] Although this definition is commonly used, it is not the only CAI definition available.[1] Currently, there is no universally accepted clinical definition of CAI. With the multitude of definitions, clinicians and researchers have a difficult time determining when a person can be classified as suffering from CAI. Even with the inconsistent criteria, the volume of research involving participants who suffer from CAI has grown exponentially over the past couple of decades. The increased literature has resulted in a general appreciation of the complexity of the condition. Recently, Hiller et al[2] proposed a model of CAI that demonstrates its complexity. The model consists of 3 unique categories under the broad umbrella definition of CAI (Table 5-1). These 3 categories (mechanical instability, perceived instability, and recurrent sprain) can exist independently or in combination with one or both of the other categories, making 7 possible subgroups. Each category includes unique impairments that may be present in individuals with CAI.

McKeon PO, Wikstrom EA, eds. *Quick Questions in Ankle Sprains: Expert Advice in Sports Medicine* (pp 25-28).

Table 5-1

Common Measures for Classifying the 3 Categories of Chronic Ankle Instability

Category of Chronic Ankle Instability		
Mechanical Instability	*Perceived Instability*	*Recurrent Ankle Sprain*
Hypermobility	Self-reported ankle instability	Ankle sprain history
Anterior drawer	Ankle-instability instrument	Number of sprains
Talar tilt	Cumberland ankle instability tool	Severity of sprain
Posterior talar glide test	Identification of functional ankle instability	Last significant sprain
Hypomobility	Self-reported ankle function	Physician visit
Dorsiflexion	Foot and ankle ability measure	
Weight-bearing lunge test	Foot and ankle outcome score	

	Functional tests:
	    Balance
	    Figure of 8
	    Lateral hop test	

Mechanical instability is the type of instability due to at least one ankle sprain that results in anatomical changes at the ankle that cause abnormal joint mechanics.[3] Mechanical instability is determined by impairments in the ankle's range of motion, namely hypermobility of the ankle joint. Most commonly, individuals with mechanical instability present with damage primarily to the anterior talofibular ligament and secondarily of the calcaneofibular ligament. These joint alterations manifest clinically as increased anterior talar glide via the anterior drawer test and increased talar inversion via the talar tilt test. Although increased laxity is the most commonly reported mechanical instability, range-of-motion deficits can also occur. Structural alignment changes after a lateral ankle sprain may cause the talus to sit more anteriorly in relation to the mortise. The abnormal placement of the talus shifts the talocrural joint axis anteriorly, resulting in diminished posterior talar glide, which presents clinically as decreased dorsiflexion range of motion.

The second category in the Hiller et al model, perceived instability, is defined on the basis of the patient's self-reported feelings of instability with no associated mechanical deficits.[2] Individuals who fit into the perceived-instability group often report a feeling of "weakness" or "looseness" in their ankle or possibly feelings of their ankle "giving way." However, clinically, these patients do not present with signs of mechanical instability. Originally, this condition was classified as "functional instability," indicating deficits with performance.[3] The shift from "functional instability" to "perceived instability" occurred because not all individuals who subjectively reported limitations actually presented with them upon evaluation. Perceived instability has been measured using various questionnaires such as the foot and ankle ability measure (FAAM) and the FAAM sports subscale, the Cumberland ankle instability tool (CAIT), and the identification of functional ankle instability (IdFAI). These questionnaires ask individuals how they feel during various activities. Individuals with perceived instability may also present with altered sensorimotor function, such as decreased lower-leg muscle strength, balance impairments, and functional deficits while running, cutting, and landing.[4] These sensorimotor impairments have been most commonly measured in research laboratories and may be difficult to detect clinically. However, several clinical tests, including balance, agility, and functional tests, have shown promise in identifying these deficits. Interestingly, the deficits observed during testing may result from fear, loss of confidence, and/or actual sensorimotor impairments.

The last category in the Hiller et al CAI model is recurrent sprain. Individuals are included within this category if they have a history of 3 or more sprains to the same ankle.[2] Upon physical assessment, individuals in this category do not present with any type of mechanical instability, and they do not report any perceived instability issues with their ankles; however, they have a history of multiple ankle sprains.

The Hiller et al CAI model does an excellent job of describing the impairments that may be present in individuals classified as having CAI. However, a question must be asked: Are these categories and subcategories of CAI actually contributing factors to the pathology or consequences of the pathology? It is currently unknown whether any of these factors, or other unexplored factors, are present in individuals prior to the initial ankle sprain predisposing them to developing CAI. Also, CAI is not determined immediately following the initial ankle sprain. Currently, there is no understanding of the time frame of development of CAI. For some, the impairments become apparent following the initial ankle sprain. For others, the classification of CAI may result from the accumulative effect of multiple ankle sprains. The classification of CAI is determined after an individual fits into one or more of the 3 categories. Potentially, the treatment and/or rehabilitation of an ankle sprain may be a critical contributing factor to the development to CAI.

CAI is a complex multifactorial condition that many people experience after an initial lateral ankle sprains. Unfortunately, the majority of evidence on CAI comes from those who have already developed the condition compared to those who never sprained an ankle. Very little evidence exists about those who sprain their ankle for the first time and then go on to develop CAI. It is not clear what factors may predispose a person to the development of CAI, but clearly, it is an issue that many patients and clinicians face. Careful study of patients with ankle sprain is critical and, most important, should capture elements of mechanical and perceived instability as well as ankle sprain recurrence.

References

1. Delahunt E, Coughlan G, Caulfield B, et al. Inclusion criteria when investigating insufficiencies in chronic ankle instability. *Med Sci Sports Exerc*. 2010;42:2106.
2. Hiller CE, Kilbreath SL, Refshauge KM. Chronic ankle instability: evolution of the model. *J Athl Train*. 2011;46:133-141.
3. Hertel J. Functional anatomy, pathomechanics, and pathophysiology of lateral ankle instability. *J Athl Train*. 2002;37:364-375.
4. Hertel J. Sensorimotor deficits with ankle sprains and chronic ankle instability. *Clin Sports Med*. 2008;27:353-370.

WHAT EFFECT DOES PROPHYLACTIC BRACING AND/OR TAPING HAVE ON REDUCING LATERAL ANKLE SPRAIN RISK?

Timothy A. McGuine, PhD, ATC

For many years, providers have had to rely on taping and bracing research that consisted of laboratory studies that detailed measures of ankle biomechanics and athletic performance as proxy measures of efficacy rather than prospective trials conducted in athletic populations.

Despite its widespread use, ankle taping has not been well studied prospectively in athlete populations. The limited data do show that athletes with a history of previous injury benefited from prophylactic ankle taping. On the other hand, several large well-controlled studies have reported that both semirigid and lace-up braces are effective in reducing the incidence of ankle sprains in adolescent and college-age athletes. Noteworthy are the findings that bracing reduced the risk of injury in athletes without a previous injury and did not increase the risk for other lower-extremity injuries.

There is good evidence to support the use of prophylactic bracing to prevent ankle sprains. Less clear is the evidence to support the use of prophylactic taping. Providers should consider the efficacy and attributes of taping and bracing within the context of a specific athletes to determine which method of external support to use.

McKeon PO, Wikstrom EA, eds. *Quick Questions in Ankle Sprains: Expert Advice in Sports Medicine* (pp 29-33).
© 2015 SLACK Incorporated.

Background

Prophylactic taping and bracing have been used extensively by sports medicine providers for decades to prevent ankle sprain injuries in youth, adolescent, and adult competitive and recreational athletes. While no numbers actually exist to document the use of prophylactic ankle support, it is safe to assume that sports medicine providers use these measures more than any other injury-prevention mechanism.

Historically, tape and braces were used to provide a mechanism to limit excessive foot and ankle motion. In recent years, sports medicine providers have often cited the growing body of thought that these external support measures enhance neuromuscular function through tactile stimulation equal to or greater than an effective mechanical restriction of foot and ankle motion.[1]

Despite the widespread use of taping and bracing to prevent ankle sprains, the question often posed by many sports medicine providers is simply this: Will taping or bracing actually prevent ankle sprains in my athletes? This may seem to be a straightforward question, but in reality, it can best be answered in the context of secondary questions that include the following: (1) Why consider taping or bracing? (2) Are there advantages/disadvantages of these methods? (3) Will athletes without any history of ankle sprain benefit from taping or bracing? (4) Will taping or bracing increase the risk for other injuries to the knee or lower leg?

Attributes of Taping and Bracing

The primary rationale for using taping or bracing to prevent ankle sprains is that their preventive effect is noticed immediately when used by an athlete. On the other hand, traditional lower-leg neuromuscular training programs develop their protective effect over an 8- to 10-week time period.[1] Taping and bracing both offer specific advantages and disadvantages. The main advantage for ankle tape is that it can be tailored to the specific shape of an athlete's lower leg, ankle, and foot, providing appropriate and varying support as necessary for the athlete. The disadvantages to taping include (1) a traditional tape job, using anchor strips, stirrups, heel locks, and figure eights, requires the time and expertise of a trained provider, (2) it loosens in as little as 20 to 30 minutes of activity, possibly negating some of its protective effect, and (3) it costs several dollars per application, translating to several hundred dollars spent per ankle over an entire sport season.

The advantages of braces include the facts that they can be (1) applied by the athletes themselves, (2) tightened periodically throughout the session to provide continuous support to the ankle, and (3) reused throughout the entire season. A disadvantage to bracing is that braces are essentially designed to fit every ankle in the same manner. This can translate to various levels of tension, support, and stress depending on an athlete's specific lower-leg, ankle, and foot shape.

Evidence

The majority of research supporting the effectiveness of taping and bracing to prevent ankle sprains actually consists of small laboratory studies that detail measures of ankle joint motion, lower-limb biomechanics, and athletic performance in collegiate and adult subjects.[2] A number of studies reported the efficacy of both methods in preventing recurrent ankle sprains in recently injured subjects or measured their effectiveness prophylactically in adult athletes.[1,2] While these studies do provide useful information, they often do not offer the level of evidence sports medicine providers need to fully evaluate their effectiveness in a young athlete population. There are, however, a limited number of prospective studies that have reported the effect that prophylactic taping or bracing has on reducing the incidence of ankle sprains in young athlete populations.

Taping

Despite the widespread use of prophylactic ankle taping, only one large randomized controlled trial of collegiate intramural basketball players supports the use of a traditional taping method (applying anchor strips, stirrups, heel locks, and figure eights) to prevent ankle sprains. Garrick and Requa[3] reported that nontaped college-aged intramural basketball players were twice as likely to sustain an ankle sprain than the taped subjects while competing. The protective effect was most pronounced in players with a history of previous ankle injury, with the numbers needed to treat (NNT) equal to 26 versus subjects with no previous history (NNT = 143). The NNT is the expected number of athletes a clinician would need to treat to prevent one injury and can be used to gauge the benefit of a treatment. The limited taping evidence indicates that, while prophylactic taping reduced the risk of ankle sprains, those with a history of ankle sprains benefited greatly compared to those with no history.

Unfortunately, the limited evidence available indicates that there is a need for well-designed randomized clinical trials to examine the effect of traditional ankle taping on the incidence of ankle sprains. Needed as well are well-controlled trials that compare the effectiveness of taping to bracing methods in actual athletic populations over an entire season of multiple practice and competition sessions.

Bracing

Compared to taping, there is considerably more evidence to support the use of bracing to prevent ankle sprains. One notable well-controlled study by Sitler et al[4] illustrated the effectiveness of semirigid (hard plastic) braces in preventing ankle sprains. Military cadets not wearing braces were 3 times more likely to sustain an ankle sprain while participating in intramural basketball. The protective effect was most pronounced in players with a previous history of ankle sprain (NNT = 18) compared to subjects with a previous injury (NNT = 39). The authors also reported that the incidence of knee injuries was not affected by wearing the braces. In comparison to the taping evidence, bracing appears to be prophylactically beneficial for those with and without a history of ankle sprains.

In most athletic populations, prophylactic bracing involves using less rigid lace-up braces rather than the semirigid braces shown to be effective in collegiate and adult settings. Two recent large randomized trials studies reported on the effectiveness of lace-up ankle braces in high school basketball[5] and football[6] players. Basketball players not wearing braces were 3 times more likely to sustain an injury than braced subjects, while football players not wearing braces were twice as likely to sustain an ankle sprain than the players wearing braces. In basketball players, the NNT was 15, while the NNT in football players was 29. Unlike the previous studies, the braces were effective for players both with and without a history of previous ankle sprains. Also noteworthy is the finding that the risk for sustaining acute knee and other leg injuries was not increased in subjects wearing the lace-up braces.

Conclusion

There is good evidence to support the use of prophylactic bracing to prevent ankle sprains. Less clear is the evidence to support the widespread use of prophylactic taping. Both ankle taping and semirigid bracing seem to be more effective for athletes with a previous history of ankle sprain. On the other hand, lace-up braces reduced the incidence of ankle sprains in players with and without a previous injury.

Athletes using prophylactic taping or bracing do not have an increased risk of knee or other leg injuries. Sports medicine providers need to consider the efficacy and attributes of both methods within the context of a specific athlete's needs to determine which method to implement.

References

1. Verhagen E, Bay K. Optimising ankle sprain prevention: a critical review and practical appraisal of literature. *Br J Sports Med.* 2010;1082-1088.
2. Kaminski TW, Hertel J, Amendola N, et. al. National Athletic Trainers' Association position statement: conservative management and prevention of ankle sprains in athletes. *J Athl Train.* 2013;48:528-545.
3. Garrick JG, Requa RK. Role of external support in the prevention of ankle sprains. *Med Sci Sports.* 1973;5:200-203.
4. Sitler M, Ryan J, Wheeler B, et al. The efficacy of a semi-rigid ankle stabilizer to reduce acute ankle injuries in basketball: a randomized clinical study at West Point. *Am J Sports Med.* 1994;22:454–461.
5. McGuine TA, Brooks A, Hetzel S. The effect of lace-up ankle braces on injury rates in high school basketball players. *Am J Sports Med.* 2011;39:1840-1848.
6. McGuine TA, Hetzel S, Wilson J, Brooks A. The effect of lace-up ankle braces on injury rates in high school football players. *Am J Sports Med.* 2012;40:49-57.

To What Extent Does Ankle Bracing or Taping Impair Functional Performance?

Mitchell L. Cordova, PhD, ATC, FNATA, FACSM

Ankle injuries, specifically lateral ankle sprains, remain the most common injuries that occur in sports and recreational activity. Because of the high incidence of ankle injuries in sport, the use of external ankle supports has been advocated by certified athletic trainers and other sports medicine professionals over many decades to prevent ankle injuries from occurring and to limit the frequency with which ankle sprains recur.

Many different types of external ankle supports exist on the market today. These devices vary from simple lace-up style braces that are constructed of soft nylon and polyester materials to more sophisticated semirigid designs that use anatomical hinges and plastic polymer materials that provide more structural rigidity (Figure 7-1). In addition to the commercially available external ankle supports, the use of adhesive taping has historically been the choice of certified athletic trainers in helping prevent ankle injuries. Ankle taping, lace-up style braces, and semirigid orthoses are used in an effort to prevent ankle injuries, as well as to stabilize patients who suffer from chronic ankle instability. Ankle bracing and taping have been shown to reduce ankle injury and injury frequency rates principally because of the mechanical support offered by these devices.[1,2] The primary function of many

McKeon PO, Wikstrom EA, eds. *Quick Questions in Ankle Sprains: Expert Advice in Sports Medicine* (pp 35-40).
© 2015 SLACK Incorporated.

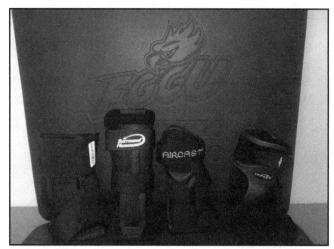

Figure 7-1. Comparison of different types of lace-up, semi-rigid, and hybrid lace-up and semirigid external ankle support (from left to right): DonJoy Stabilizing Speed Pro (lace-up), DonJoy Surround Foam (semirigid), Aircast Airsport (lace-up and semirigid hybrid), and DonJoy Velocity ES (semirigid with hinged sole plate).

of the external ankle supports used today is to restrict frontal plane movement of the subtalar joint while also providing stabilization to the talocrural and distal tibiofubular articulations.[3]

The primary role of external ankle supports is to mechanically limit joint range of motion in the sagittal and frontal planes. Because certain types of external ankle supports can be very restrictive depending on the materials of which they are composed (ie, semirigid orthoses) and how tightly they are applied (ie, adhesive tape), many sports medicine practitioners have surmised that the restrictions being placed on the foot and ankle joint motion translate into diminished lower-extremity functional performance of the athlete. These concerns have ranged from the athlete not being able to run as fast, to not being able to jump as high, or to not being able to make quick changes in different directions.[4] Of all the empirical data that exist in the literature surrounding the use of external ankle support, the impact that ankle bracing and taping have on functional performance is probably most important. Another important aspect that must not be overlooked is the athlete's perception of whether external ankle support will hinder his or her performance—even if the preponderance of data in the literature suggest that it does not. Additionally, the type of athlete and the sport played may also affect the athlete's perception of whether external ankle support will impede performance. For example, a soccer player not only has to run fast, demonstrate great agility, and jump for balls, but he or she also has to handle the ball with great finesse and "touch." In this case, the soccer player may view the use of external ankle support as "too bulky" for the foot, thereby decreasing his or her sensitivity in connection to the soccer ball, even though lower-extremity functional performance is not affected. Conversely, a basketball player who also needs to run fast, demonstrate great agility, and jump high throughout the course of the game may perceive external ankle support to be protective and therefore more helpful in performing the sport. Ultimately, even though ankle taping and bracing have been shown to be beneficial in preventing ankle injuries, athletes will avoid wearing such an appliance if they perceive that it hinders their athletic performance.

Several investigations over the past 45 years have examined the influence of external ankle support on sprint speed, agility, and vertical jump height in an attempt to answer the question that many certified athletic trainers and sports medicine practitioners have often thought to ask: does the benefit of ankle stabilization come with a level of compromise that manifests into decreased functional performance ability? The general effectiveness of ankle bracing and taping on lower-extremity functional performance has been discussed in 2 previous extensive narrative reviews[3,5] and comprehensively examined in a meta-analysis, from which a true estimate of the effects strongly suggests that external ankle stabilizers *do not* negatively affect running speed, agility, or vertical jump height in a substantial manner. A synthesis of the effects of external ankle support on different facets of lower-extremity functional performance measures (eg, running speed, agility, and vertical jump height) follows.

Running Speed and External Ankle Support

The ability to run fast is a major component in most sports and physical activities. The type of external ankle support applied to the foot and ankle joint complex will influence the amount of sagittal plane motion restriction, thereby potentially diminishing the propulsion forces generated during running gait that ultimately contribute to overall running speed. The specific effects of different types of ankle bracing and adhesive tape application on pure sprint performance have been extensively studied, and the overall standardized effects range from trivial to a small decrement.[4] Collectively, the actual transformation of these effects represents a 1% decrease in running speed (Table 7-1). The question that often begs to be answered is this: Do these effects translate into real functional differences? If you consider a running back performing a timed 40-yard sprint in 4.5 seconds, a 1% decrease with the application of an ankle brace would add .045 seconds, resulting in an overall time of 4.55 seconds. One would surmise that this decrease in speed for the same player in a game situation would be hardly noticeable, even for an elite athlete.

Table 7-1

Meta-Analyzed Standardized Effect Sizes for the Influence of 3 Different Classifications of External Ankle Support on 3 Primary Functional Performance Measures

	External Ankle Support Type		
Outcome Measure	*Tape*	*Lace-up*	*Semirigid*
Running speed	-0.14 ± 0.00 (1%)	-0.22 ± 0.00 (1%)	-0.10 ± 0.30 (1%)
Agility speed	-0.01 ± 0.00 (0.1%)	0.03 ± 0.00 (0.2%)	0.05 ± 0.18 (0.4%)
Vertical jump height	-0.14 ± 0.24 (1%)	-0.04 ± 0.00 (1%)	-0.07 ± 0.00 (1%)

Data are mean ± true between-effect SD, with percent decrease in performance test in parentheses.

Adapted with permission from Lippincott Williams & Wilkins and Wilkins/Wolters Kluwer Health: *Medicine and Science in Sports and Exercise.*[4]

There is convincing evidence in the literature indicating that the application of external ankle support does not limit running speed or sprint performance.

Agility Performance and External Ankle Support

Similar to running speed and sprint performance, agility also represents a complex movement pattern that is essential to many sports and physical activities. Many research investigations have employed different types of testing protocols in an effort to challenge the coordination and speed of subjects simulating agility patterns used in different types of sports. These agility protocols typically require rapid changes in movement direction in which phases of acceleration and deceleration are combined (eg, running a figure 8 around cones, SEMO agility test, and shuttle run). When assessing the effects of adhesive tape, lace-up style ankle braces, and semirigid ankle bracing on agility speed, the type of support may also influence performance during an agility test similar to what is observed with running speed. The specific effects of adhesive tape and different types of external ankle support on agility performance have also been extensively examined. The results of this work have demonstrated, collectively, that the overall influence of these devices is trivial.[4] When establishing the functional manifestation of these trivial effects, it has been established that, overall the application of an external ankle support results in a performance decrease of 0.4% or less (see Table 7-1). For example, a women's volleyball player performing a figure-8 cone course in 35 seconds or less without ankle bracing or taping would add up to 0.14 seconds to her overall time with the use of external ankle support. Similar to sprint performance, it is highly unlikely that this decrease in agility speed would translate into a clinically meaningful detrimental effect. Of the 3 most highly assessed lower-extremity functional performance tests investigated in the literature, the evidence strongly indicates that external ankle support does not hinder agility speed.

Vertical Jump Height and External Ankle Support

When performing a vertical jump or a jump that requires vertical and anterior projection of the body, the total range of motion available at the talocrural joint will influence the height and length obtained during the jump because of the rapid eccentric loading of the gastrocnemius-soleus musculature followed by concentric contraction of the same muscle group. The mechanical design of an externally applied ankle brace or the ankle tape application technique will influence how much talocrural joint motion is available. For example, a lace-up style ankle brace and the traditional basketweave ankle-taping technique may restrict the extremes of sagittal plane motion, which could decrease the amount of height obtained during a vertical jump, whereas a semirigid stirrup type appliance allows for greater sagittal plane motion regardless of the type of jump protocol used.[3] Collectively, all 3 categories of external ankle support may negatively influence vertical jump height obtained, but these effects are trivial. Of these effects, it is not surprising that the application of adhesive tape has the greatest negative impact on vertical jump performance, although as stated earlier, this effect is trivial.[4] The semirigid and lace-up style ankle braces may negatively influence vertical jump height similarly, but these effects are even smaller than that observed with ankle taping (see Table 7-1). Similar to its effect on sprint performance, external ankle support negatively affects vertical jump height by 1%. For athletes whose sports necessitate the ability to jump high (eg, volleyball or basketball), a 1% decrease would translate into an overall decrease of 0.76 cm (0.3 inches) to the jump. Similar to its effect on running speed, there is convincing evidence in the literature that external ankle support does not hinder vertical jump performance.

Conclusion

The effects of external ankle support on lower-extremity functional performance measures have been extensively studied with running speed, agility, and vertical jump as the primary dependent variables. The functional range of motion permitted at the ankle and foot joint complex with the application of an external ankle support is established by the structure, design, and materials that make up the support. The results from multiple narrative literature reviews[3,5] and from a very extensive meta-analysis[4] suggest that external ankle support has virtually no negative effect on running speed, agility speed, or vertical jump ability. The use of external ankle support is effective in preventing acute and chronic ankle injury while not hindering functional performance.

References

1. Surve I, Schwellnus MP, Noakes T, Lombard C. A fivefold reduction in the incidence of recurrent ankle sprains in soccer players using the sport-stirrup orthosis. *Am J Sports Med.* 1994;12:601-606.
2. Sitler M, Ryan J, Wheeler B, et al. The efficacy of a semirigid ankle stabilizer to reduce acute ankle injuries in basketball: a randomized clinical study at West Point. *Am J Sports Med.* 1994;12:454-461.
3. Cordova ML, Ingersoll CD, Palmieri RP. Efficacy of prophylactic ankle support: an experimental perspective. *J Athl Train.* 2002;37:446-457.
4. Cordova ML, Scott BD, Ingersoll CD, LeBlanc MJ. The effects of prophylactic ankle support on lower extremity functional performance: a meta-analysis. *Med Sci Sports Exerc.* 2005;37:635-641.
5. Bot SD, van Mechelen W. The effect of ankle bracing on athletic performance. *Sports Med.* 1999;27:171-178.

WHAT TYPES OF PREVENTIVE EXERCISES COULD HELP REDUCE AN ATHLETE'S RISK OF SUFFERING A LATERAL ANKLE SPRAIN?

Evert Verhagen, PhD, FECSS

Prophylactic taping, braces, high-top shoes, and neuromuscular training (NMT) have all been postulated as preventive measures against ankle sprains. Many studies have been published in which the preventive effects against ankle sprains of each of these measures have been described. According to the scientific literature, the prevention of ankle sprains with external measures that aim to limit ankle range of motion (ie, brace or tape) are equally effective as the use of NMT. Both types of measures have been linked to a 50% reduction of the risk of sustaining an ankle sprain. However, a preventive effect has been shown over consecutive years for athletes with a previous injury.[1]

Individuals who sustain an ankle sprain have a twofold risk of reinjury up to 2 years after injury. This increased injury risk after an initial ankle sprain is generally thought to be the result of a combined proprioceptive, strength, and range-of-motion (ROM) impairment of the ankle after trauma. Partly on the basis of this rationale, NMT is widely used for rehabilitation after an ankle sprain. NMT, which is roughly defined as a combination of strength, flexibility, and proprioceptive exercises, is thought to improve ankle function by re-establishing and strengthening the protective reflexes of the ankle.

McKeon PO, Wikstrom E, eds. *Quick Questions in Ankle Sprains: Expert Advice in Sports Medicine* (pp 41-44).

External Measures vs Exercise

It has been well described in the literature that external measures, especially semirigid bracing, achieve a great preventive effect and that such measures are an excellent primary prevention strategy (ie, preventing first-time ankle sprains). However, external measures are suggested to only protect the ankle by limiting the maximal ankle movement as opposed to restrengthening and retraining the ankle. Additionally, external measures work only when actually applied during participation in sports, whereas NMT provides a sustainable effect. External measures, as such, do not provide the added benefit of NMT. Moreover, NMT has not only been proven to be an effective and cost-effective preventive measure but has also been linked to a reduction in residual ankle sprain complaints such as pain and instability. As such, NMT is considered the secondary preventive measure of choice.

Added use of external measures to support the ankle may be implemented for patients who are at increased risk for subsequent injury and thus require special considerations, especially for the subgroup with a history of previous injury or episodes of ankle instability.[2] In this subgroup, subsequent reinjury risk highly depends on (1) the type of rehabilitation employed, (2) whether the subject complied with the rehabilitation program, and (3) the quality of recovery. From this perspective, structured rehabilitation programs that include restoration of normal ankle motion, strengthening, and restoration of neuromuscular control and proprioception of the ankle complex should be advocated. Until function is completely normal, patients should be urged to make use of either ankle taping or a brace for external support.

Postrehabilitation Phase

A number of NMT programs to be used after the rehabilitative phase have been described. Some programs are sports or context specific, and within the literature, effective programs have been described for, among others, handball, soccer, volleyball, and basketball.[3] The reported effectiveness of such programs in reducing ankle sprain reinjury risk ranges from a relative risk reduction of 80% to 30%. This wide range can be explained by the intensity and context of the preventive program; sport-specific and prolonged programs seem to achieve the greatest preventive effect. In part, this may be explained by the patient's adherence to the prescribed exercise scheme in these programs (see also "Patient Adherence").

Figure 8-1 depicts a universal NMT program that can be carried out individually by the patient after rehabilitation without the necessity of further supervision. There is good evidence to support this program as an effective and cost-efficient

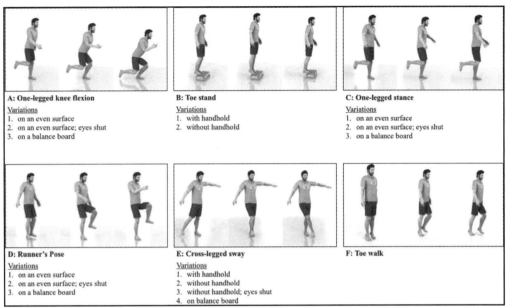

Figure 8-1. Exercises in a home-based NMT program.

Table 8-1
Exercise Scheme for the 8-Week Training Program
Training (three times per week for a period of 8 weeks)

Exercise		Week 1			Week 2			Week 3			Week 4			Week 5			Week 6			Week 7			Week 8		
		1	2	3	1	2	3	1	2	3	1	2	3	1	2	3	1	2	3	1	2	3	1	2	3
	A	1	1	1	1	1	1	1	1	2	2	2	2	2	2	2	3	3	3	3	3	3	3	3	3
	B	1	1	1	1	1	1	1	1	1	1	1	1	2	2	2	2	2	2	2	2	2	2	2	2
	C	1	1	1	1	2	2	2	2	3	3	3	3	3	3	3	3	3	3	3	3	3	3	3	3
	D	1	1	1	1	2	2	2	2	3	3	3	3	3	3	3	3	3	3	3	3	3	3	3	3
	E	1	1	1	1	1	1	2	2	2	2	2	2	3	3	3	3	4	4	4	4	4	4	4	4
	F	1	1	1	1	1	1	1	1	1	1	1	1	2	2	2	2	2	2	2	2	2	2	2	2

program after rehabilitation; it limits both the risk and severity of subsequent injury.[3] In a randomized controlled trial, the program was linked to a 35% relative risk reduction of resprains. Additionally, a subgroup analysis revealed that the program also effectively reduces reinjury severity, whereas the greatest risk reduction (75%) was established for the more severe reinjuries.

This program incorporates 3 weekly sets of simple exercises over an 8-week period (Table 8-1). There are also exercises in this NMT program to be carried out on a balance board or foam mat. If a balance board or foam mat is not available, these materials can be interchanged by other unstable surfaces (eg, a thick pillow or a mattress). Thereby, this program provides an inexpensive and accessible tool that is effective for all. To support the patient, this program is now also available as an interactive smartphone application (Ankle, available for iOS and Android) guiding the patient through the exercise scheme while providing feedback on the program's proceedings.

Patient Adherence

In order to effectively reduce the risk of an ankle injury, adherence to exercises is of utmost importance. Especially in an NMT program in which active engagement of a patient is required, program adherence is the key to success or failure. Logically, preventive programs are effective only when patients perform them and are exposed to a critical dose of the exercises. In general, it is recommended that a patient follow at least 75% of a full program, a percentage loosely based on research outcomes. One should be aware, however, that the missed exercises should not be mainly in succession (ie, perform for only 6 weeks of an 8-week program).

It is recommended that the clinician motivate and educate patients during the rehabilitation phase on the necessity of continuing NMT beyond when they return to participation. During rehabilitation, the clinician can guide the patient through exercises and build a base to encourage prolonged exercises after rehabilitation.

References

1. Verhagen E, Bay K. Optimising ankle sprain prevention: a critical review and practical appraisal of the literature. *Br J Sports Med.* 2010;44:1082–1088.
2. Fong DT-P, Hong Y, Chan L-K, et al. A systematic review on ankle injury and ankle sprain in sports. *Sports Med.* 2007;37:73–94.
3. Hupperets M, Verhagen E, Mechelen WV. Effect of unsupervised home based proprioceptive training on recurrences of ankle sprain: randomised controlled trial. *Br Med J.* 2009;339:b2684.

WHAT IS THE COMPARATIVE COST-EFFECTIVENESS OF LATERAL ANKLE SPRAIN PREVENTION STRATEGIES?

Luke Donovan, PhD, ATC and
Jay Hertel, PhD, ATC

Consequences of a lateral ankle sprain (LAS) may include time lost from sport, a high reinjury rate, a long-term decrease in physical activity, osteoarthritis, and high medical costs associated with diagnosis and treatment. Currently, there is not an up-to-date lifetime cost estimate of an LAS, but the median amount billed to an individual who reports to an emergency department in the United States with a general sprain is about $1051.00.[1] This number does not include future costs of physical therapy and health care equipment associated with treating an LAS. Due to the high incident rate and consequences of LAS, it is common for clinicians, coaches, and athletes to implement LAS-prevention strategies during their sport season. The most common strategies are ankle taping, ankle bracing, and balance-training programs. It is important to establish the cost-effectiveness for each strategy to ensure that the benefit outweighs the costs associated with them. This can be done by reviewing the literature to establish the effectiveness of each strategy, calculating the number needed to treat (NNT), and multiplying that by the estimated cost of each strategy. Overall, each strategy mentioned earlier has been found to have a similar risk reduction (50% to 80%) in terms of preventing LAS.

McKeon PO, Wikstrom EA, eds. *Quick Questions in Ankle Sprains: Expert Advice in Sports Medicine* (pp 45-49).
© 2015 SLACK Incorporated.

Ankle Taping

Ankle taping is one of the most common strategies for preventing LAS; however, there is little evidence on its effectiveness. The largest randomized controlled clinical trial (RCT) to determine the effectiveness of ankle taping for preventing ankle sprains in intramural basketball players was completed in the early 1970s.[2] Although this work by Garrick and Requa[2] should not be discredited, it is important to note that the changes in footwear, tape, and field surfaces over the past 40 years could influence their results. On the basis of Garrick and Requa's results, they found a decrease in LAS in athletes who were taped and the biggest decrease in individuals with previous LAS.

To calculate a cost estimate, the NNT was calculated, the length of the season was approximated, and the cost of tape was estimated. The NNT to prevent one LAS, regardless of sprain history, was 56. In order to prevent a recurrent LAS, 26 individuals with a history of LAS need to be treated. Finally, to prevent one LAS in individuals with no history of LAS, 143 individuals need to be treated throughout the season. An average basketball season lasts approximately 16 weeks. This approximation does not include preseason and postseason play. If we assume that most teams practice or compete 6 days/week, we can estimate 96 exposures for each person participating on the team per season. Currently, a box of 32 rolls of athletic tape costs approximately $60.45 or $1.89 per roll of tape. To calculate the cost estimate of using tape to prevent an LAS over the course of a season, we used the formula used by Olmsted et al[3]: [NNT × cost of tape (1.89) × exposures (96)]. If one roll of tape is used per person per exposure, to prevent one LAS regardless of sprain history will cost $105.84 per exposure (ie, practice or game) and $10,160.64 over the season. Furthermore, it will cost $49.14 per exposure to prevent one LAS in individuals with a history of LAS and $4717.44 over the season. Finally, to prevent one LAS in individuals with no history of LAS costs $270.27 per exposure and $25,945.92 over the season. Cost estimates of each strategy are presented in Table 9-1.

Ankle Bracing

Recently, there were 2 large RCTs that examined the effects of ankle bracing on LAS injury rates in high school football[4] and basketball players.[5] Both of these studies found a significant reduction in ankle injury rate regardless of previous LAS history. Because of the data provided from the articles, the NNT was calculated only for the entire population disregarding LAS history. In high school football players,[4] the NNT was 29 and was 15 in high school basketball players.[5]

Table 9-1

Comparative Cost Estimates Between Taping, Bracing, and Balance Programs to Prevent Lateral Ankle Sprain During Sport Based on Number Needed to Treat

	No History of Ankle Sprain			History of Ankle Sprain			Pooled Population			
	Taping	*Bracing*	*Balance*	*Taping*	*Bracing*	*Balance*	*Taping*	*Bracing*		*Balance*
								Basketball	Football	
Cost of Intervention	$1.89	$67.90	$114.45	$1.89	$67.90	$114.45	$1.89	$67.90	$67.90	$114.45
NNT	143	—	—	26	—	20	56	15	29	25
Cost per Ankle Sprain	$270.27	—	—	$49.14	—	$2289	$105.84	$1018.50	$1961.10	$2861.25
Number of Intervention Costs per Season	96	—	—	96	—	1	96	1	1	1
Total Cost per Season	$25,945.92	—	—	$4717.44	—	$2289	$10,160.64	$1018.50	$1961.10	$2861.25

Using the brace from the McGuine et al basketball study,[5] the cost of 2 McDavid 195 Ultralight ankle braces is $67.90 (Patterson Medical Holdings, Inc). To prevent one LAS in high school football using braces would cost $1961.10 and would cost $1018.50 in high school basketball. Because ankle braces are recommended to be replaced every year, these are the total costs associated with each season. Bracing across an entire season costs approximately 10% that of taping and results in a more effective prevention of ankle sprains.

Balance Training

Balance-training programs are thought to improve athletic performance and decrease multiple types of injuries. These programs are appealing, because individuals do not wear extra equipment, and programs can be implemented into routine prepractice warm-ups. A study by Verhagen et al[6] examined the effects of balance training on injury rates in young adult volleyball players. The volleyball teams in the intervention group received 5 wobble boards and an instructional balance-training video. In addition to the video, coaches were provided progression instructions by a physiotherapist. During their warm-up, each person completed balance training using the wobble board. Incorporating balance exercises in the daily warm-up significantly decreased the rate of LAS in individuals with a previous history of LAS.[6] The NNT, regardless of sprain history, was 25 and the NNT to prevent one LAS in those with a previous history of LAS was 20.[6] The NNT in individuals with no history of LAS could not be calculated with the data provided.

Cost estimates for balance-training programs vary on the basis of implementation and equipment. For example, Verhagen et al[6] used one training period session with a physical therapist, an instructional video, and wobble boards. In the United States, the direct cost of a 15-minute neuromuscular training session with a sports medicine professional is about $37.50 and a wobble board is about $76.95 (Patterson Medical Holdings, Inc). On the basis of Verhagen et al[6] NNT, if individuals chose to learn a balance program from a sports medicine professional, purchase their own wobble board, and complete the program at home, it would cost $2861.25 to prevent one LAS from occurring regardless of past LAS history. It would cost $2289 to prevent one LAS from occurring if only the individuals with previous injury completed the program. If the program was completed by a team approach, each of these estimated costs would be at least 50% lower because of the need to buy fewer wobble boards. In addition, the wobble boards can be used each year, making the long-term cost of balance-training programs almost $0 as long as a person affiliated with the team is able to provide instructions. This is an important consideration when comparing these NNT and cost findings to those of ankle taping and bracing, which require yearly purchases of materials.

Balance training has the lowest long-term costs associated with preventing LAS if a team-based approach is used. As far as effectiveness, bracing has been shown to decrease LAS in individuals with and without previous history of ankle injury,[4,5] whereas balance programs[6] and taping[2] seem to best decrease LAS in individuals with previous injury. Therefore, it is recommended to implement a long-term balance-training program for individuals with a history of LAS and use ankle bracing in individuals with no previous ankle injury when trying to prevent LAS. Caution should be advised in interpreting these results, because each study examined a different population in terms of age and sport. In addition, no large RCTs exist for the comparative prophylactic effectiveness of taping, bracing, and balance programs or the summative effect when used in conjunction with each other. Most important, it is clear from this evidence that the long-term treatment costs of ankle sprains, in addition to the emergency department costs discussed earlier, would be far greater than the cost associated with the prophylactic benefits of bracing and balance training.

References

1. Caldwell N, Srebotnjak T, Wang T, Hsia R. "How much will I get charged for this?" Patient charges for top ten diagnoses in the emergency department. *PLoS One.* 2013;8:e55491.
2. Garrick JG, Requa RK. Role of external support in the prevention of ankle sprains. *Med Sci Sports.* 1973;5:200-203.
3. Olmsted LC, Vela LI, Denegar CR, Hertel J. Prophylactic ankle taping and bracing: a numbers-needed-to-treat and cost-benefit analysis. *J Athl Train.* 2004;39:95.
4. McGuine TA, Hetzel S, Wilson J, Brooks A. The effect of lace-up ankle braces on injury rates in high school football players. *Am J Sports Med.* 2012;40:49-57.
5. McGuine TA, Brooks A, Hetzel S. The effect of lace-up ankle braces on injury rates in high school basketball players. *Am J Sports Med.* 2011;39:1840-1848.
6. Verhagen E, Van Tulder M, Van Der Beek A, Bouter L, Van Mechelen W. An economic evaluation of a proprioceptive balance board training programme for the prevention of ankle sprains in volleyball. *Br J Sports Med.* 2005;39:111.

SECTION II

DIAGNOSIS

HOW AND WHY
ARE ANKLE SPRAINS GRADED?

Matthew Stewart, PT, FACP

Sprains of the lateral ankle ligaments are one of the most common injuries in patients who present to sports medicine facilities. The fact that they are so prevalent has led to the belief that they are, in essence, benign injuries, and the phrase "oh, it's just a sprain" is commonplace. However, it is evident that they are mostly not benign, with up to 40% of people still having problems with their ankles 2 years after injury.[1] This can be attributed in part to a combination of incorrect diagnosis, underestimating the extent of initial injury, and inadequate rehabilitation.

Grading the extent of initial injury in the clinic is often described as subjective and unreliable.[2] This occurs because of the lack of a universally recognized standard grading system. A multitude of systems are in use and are based on findings such as the following:

- Anatomical damage
- Clinical presentation, including swelling, pain, and functional loss
- Ligamentous stability
- Mechanism of injury
- Combinations of all of the above

Overlapping nomenclature between grading scales (ie, most use a variation of grades 1 to 3) leads to confusion and reduces reliability. Furthermore, in ankle

McKeon PO, Wikstrom EA, eds. *Quick Questions in
Ankle Sprains: Expert Advice in Sports Medicine* (pp 53-57).
© 2015 SLACK Incorporated.

sprain clinical research, investigators often do not stipulate which grading scale is used for their inclusion and exclusion criteria for patients with ankle sprain. Often, it may simply be stated that patients with a particular grade (ie, grade 2 ankle sprains) were recruited and included in the study, but there can be substantial differences between what a grade 2 injury is across the different scales.

Why Are Ankle Sprains Graded?

General labeling of "just a sprain" indicates a general one-size-fits-all rehabilitation plan, which has undoubtedly contributed to the poor outcomes and high levels of disability persisting 12 to 24 months after lateral ligament injury. Time frames for injury healing are often highly underestimated without consideration for the extent of joint damage that occurred as a result of an ankle sprain. By attempting to specifically subcategorize the extent of injury (ie, grade it), a more specific and targeted rehabilitation plan can be undertaken. Being able to group patients consistently on the basis of similar injury characteristics and profiles could markedly improve what we know about ankle sprain outcomes and enhance our ability to reduce high rates of associated long-term disability.

Grading ankle sprains allows for more accurate estimations of prognosis, identification of contraindications, and enables better postinjury rehabilitation planning. This enables the formulation of rehabilitation time frames for the commencement of hopping, running, and eventual return to sport.

Detection of high-degree damage dictates that greater postinjury protection is required for tissues to repair, both in type of protection provided (eg, bracing vs taping) and duration of its use. Additionally, functional exercises need to progress more slowly, allowing adequate time for ligament repair before advanced loading. Conversely, making no attempt to grade the injury can cause an underestimate of damage, which can lead to an inappropriate rehabilitation plan that does not allow sufficient tissue repair, potentially leading to mechanical instability and persisting disability.

Grading ankle sprains reliably can potentially give clinicians insight into who goes on to develop chronic ankle instability. The current inconsistencies within the variety of ankle sprain grading scales make it unclear what type of ankle sprains lead patients to be more at risk of developing recurrent issues.

How Should Ankle Sprains Be Graded?

A major difficulty in the process of determining the grade of injury can be an overreliance on clinical stress tests (Figure 10-1). Used in isolation, they have been

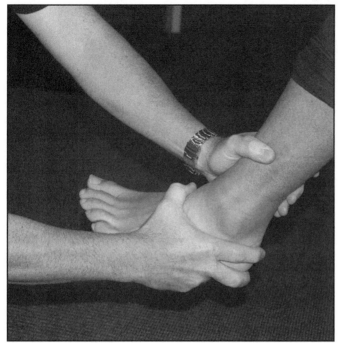

Figure 10-1. The anterior drawer test.

reported to be unreliable because of individual differences in tissue properties and ligament orientation as well as variation in forces applied by clinicians and the joint position in which the tests are performed.[2] In the acute setting, this is further complicated by diffuse pain on palpation, and it can be difficult to gauge if swelling is edema or hematoma.[3]

It has been demonstrated that delaying definitive physical examination by 4 to 5 days and evaluating clinical stress tests in combination with other physical examination findings greatly improves the accuracy of diagnosis and helps determine the extent of ligament damage.[3] Pain on specific palpation, magnitude of swelling, presence or absence of lateral hematoma (discoloration), and detectable laxity compared to the other side all build a more accurate clinical picture of the extent of injury. This allows for specific grading, which can then guide the subsequent postinjury rehabilitation.

Additionally, the choice of grading system is important. Grading systems based on intact, partial, or complete rupture are suited to single ligaments (ie, knee medial collateral ligament). This is not practical for the lateral ligament complex of the ankle, because it requires grading each individual component. It is said to be easier and more reliable to differentiate between a damaged anterior talofibular ligament (ATFL) and a combined injury to the ATFL and calcaneofibular ligament (CFL) than differentiating between an intact ATFL and a ruptured ATFL,[4] which becomes problematic when one is looking to grade an injury to the AFTL as

Table 10-1
Grading System for Lateral Ligament Injuries

No-ligament injury	Minimal amount of swelling
	No lateral discoloration
	No pain on palpation of ATFL
	No pain on palpation of CFL
	Negative ADT
	Negative IST
Single-ligament injury	Moderate amount of swelling
	Lateral hematoma
	Pain on palpation of ATFL
	No pain on palpation of CFL
	Positive ADT
	Negative IST
Double-ligament injury	Large amount of swelling
	Lateral hematoma
	Pain on palpation of ATFL
	Pain on palpation of CFL
	Positive ADT
	Positive IST

a grade 2 partial rupture. Avoiding systems that use numerical grades 1, 2, and 3 is recommended to reduce confusion between examiners and across different systems.

There is a practical system for clinical use that has 3 lateral ankle sprain classifications: no-ligament, single-ligament, or double-ligament injury.[5] On days 4 to 5 after injury under this system (Table 10-1), a no-ligament injury is characterized by minimal swelling, no pain on palpation of the ATFL or CFL, negative anterior drawer test (ADT), and negative inversion stress test (IST). This indicates intact lateral ligaments. A single-ligament injury is characterized by moderate swelling, lateral hematoma, and pain on palpation of the ATFL but not on palpation of the CFL, with positive ADT and negative IST results. This indicates a rupture, either partial or complete, of the ATFL. A double-ligament injury is characterized by significant swelling, lateral hematoma, and pain on palpation of both the ATFL and CFL in conjunction with positive ADT and positive IST results. This indicates either partial or complete ruptures involving both the ATFL and CFL. This system is less subjective and avoids the confusion associated with numerical grading scales; however, it is yet to be correlated against surgical or imaging findings. This evidence would greatly strengthen the rating system.

Conclusion

It is inadequate to label injuries to the lateral ligaments as "just a sprain." The goal should be to make a specific determination of the extent of ligament damage. This enables a better estimate of prognosis and the development of an individual rehabilitation plan. Improving the accuracy of ankle sprain grading requires a universal standardized grading scale, which currently does not exist. In the absence of a globally recognized system, avoiding the multitude of systems that use numerical grades is recommended. The magnitude of overlap within and between these scales can be confusing and reduce reliability. The grading system outlined in this chapter, while not perfect, is less subjective and can provide greater clarity in determining the extent of ligament damage in the clinical setting.

References

1. Gerber JP, Williams GN, Scoville CR, Arciero RA, Taylor DC. Persistent disability associated with ankle sprains: a prospective examination of an athletic population. *Foot Ankle Int*. 1998;19:653-660.
2. Fujii T, Luo Z, Kitaoka H, An K. The manual stress test may not be sufficient to differentiate ankle ligament injuries. *Clin Biomech*. 2000;15:619-623.
3. Van Dijk CN, Lim LS, Bossuyt PM, Marti RK. Physical examination is sufficient for the diagnosis of sprained ankles. *J Bone Joint Surg*. 1996;78-B:958-962.
4. Bahr R, Pena F, Shine J, et al. Mechanics of the anterior drawer and the talar tilt tests. *Acta Orthop Scand*. 1997;68:435-441.
5. Black H, Brand R, Eichelberger M. An improved technique for the evaluation of ligamentous injury in severe ankle sprains. *Am J Sports Med*. 1978;6:275-282.

WHAT ARE THE DIFFERENCES IN KEY CLINICAL FEATURES AMONG SYNDESMOTIC, MEDIAL, AND LATERAL ANKLE SPRAINS?

Thomas W. Kaminski, PhD, ATC, FNATA, FACSM
and Eric Nussbaum, MEd, ATC, LAT

Sports health care professionals see a plethora of acute injuries, none more common than the ankle sprain. Ankle sprains affect athletes of all ages and sporting activities, with sports that involve landing, jumping, cutting, and quick explosive actions having among the highest incidences of sprains. As clinicians, it is important to be able to distinguish between the key clinical features related to lateral, medial, and syndesmotic ankle sprains.

Lateral (inversion) ankle sprains account for the majority of all sprains to the ankle (80% to 90%) and result in damage to the lateral ligament structures (anterior talofibular, calcaneofibular, and posterior talofibular ligaments). Although most ankle sprains do not involve fractures to the surrounding bones, clinicians should nonetheless use the Ottawa ankle rules to rule out fractures.[1] Any gross deformities or abnormalities should be a red flag and justify immediate transport for follow-up diagnostic imaging. Clinicians should also consider the modifiable and nonmodifiable risk factors discussed in Questions 3 and 4 of this book. Key indicators from a clinical standpoint include tenderness over the lateral ligament structures and swelling localized to the lateral side of the ankle. More severe lateral ankle sprains

McKeon PO, Wikstrom EA, eds. *Quick Questions in
Ankle Sprains: Expert Advice in Sports Medicine* (pp 59-62).

will be distinguished by the inability of the patient to bear weight or disability by an antalgic gait, patients reporting hearing a "pop" or "snap" associated with the injury mechanism, and excessive lateral ankle joint pain, with associated positive stress tests (anterior drawer, talar tilt). Ecchymosis may not be present until 3 to 4 days after injury.

Medial (eversion) ankle sprains are a rare occurrence and account for only a small percentage (5% to 10%) of ankle sprain episodes. Bony and ligamentous anatomy account for the major differences between lateral and medial ankle sprain mechanisms and incidence rates. However, medial ankle sprains tend to be more severe and debilitating than their lateral sprain counterparts. Key distinguishing clinical features include inability of the patient to bear weight or disability by an antalgic gait, exquisite pain over the course of the deltoid ligament below the medial malleolus, and pain associated with both adduction and abduction movements of the foot. The talar tilt test may be provocative and cause pain. Unlike lateral ankle sprains, swelling associated with medial ankle sprains is usually more diffuse and less intense. Severe eversion sprains can produce significant medial joint instability, resulting in excessive foot pronation and external rotation of the lower leg ("fallen arch"). Additionally, clinicians should have a high level of suspicion for an avulsion fracture of the distal medial malleolus because of the high-level eversion forces attributed to medial sprains. In these cases, a clinician should order a radiographic evaluation.

Syndesmotic ankle sprains that demonstrate tenderness between the medial and lateral malleoli indicate potential damage to the distal tibiofibular syndesmosis and are often referred to as "high ankle sprains." In the literature, syndesmotic sprains of the ankle account for 1% to 17% of all ankle sprains, but in populations involved in sporting activities, the incidence may be much higher.[2] Syndesmotic ankle sprains seem to be diagnosed at an increasing rate because of improved recognition and differentiation between traditional ankle sprains.[3] Injury can disrupt one or all of the syndesmotic ligaments and create pain that radiates proximally above the ankle joint proper. The bones of the lower leg are held together tightly by the ligaments of the syndesmosis, which allows the tibia and fibula to act like a wrench gripping the talus. Injury to the ligaments of the syndesmosis may create widening of the joint, which results in a decreased ability for this "wrench" to "grip the nut." The anterior inferior tibiofibular ligament is the most commonly injured ligament, whereas the interosseous ligament is the strongest ligament of the syndesmosis and less involved. Syndesmotic ankle sprains most commonly occur with the mechanism of hyperdorsiflexion and pronation, but these sprains can also accompany the traditional mechanisms associated with lateral ankle sprains.[4] Injuries that involve inversion mechanisms are frequently associated with rotation, a prior history of ankle sprain, or with those ankles that have a greater degree of lateral laxity. Key

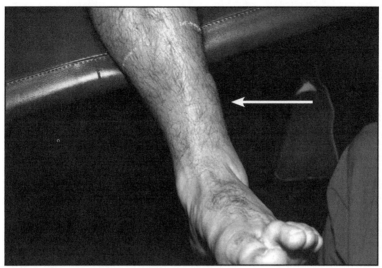

Figure 11-1. Syndesmotic ankle sprain. Note the excessive swelling proximal to the ankle joint (arrow).

clinical features include inability to bear weight, gait modification by externally rotating the foot, or walking more flat footed, because loaded dorsiflexion is often challenging and creates pain. Swelling may be a distinctive feature associated with syndesmotic sprains (Figure 11-1). Syndesmotic injury may be progressive in nature, resulting in multidirectional instability, functional disability, chronic pain, heterotopic ossification, recurrent lateral sprains, and a complaint of not being able to "push off."[5] Because of the anatomical and biomechanical importance of the syndesmosis, syndesmotic ankle sprains should not be underestimated. If the key signs and symptoms of syndesmotic ankle sprains are present in a patient, appropriate rest and recovery are essential for preventing injury recurrence.

Clinicians need to accurately and efficiently assess ankle sprains and initiate management strategies immediately after injury. Having the ability to differentiate subtle features between lateral, medial, and syndesmotic sprains can aid in a quicker recovery on the part of the patient. Point tenderness on palpation of specific ligamentous structures, as well as the inability to bear weight are key clinical features (Table 11-1).

Table 11-1		
Key Clinical Features of the Three Types of Ankle Sprains		
Lateral Ankle Sprain	**Medial Ankle Sprain**	**Syndesmotic Ankle Sprain**
Lateral ligament tenderness	Medial ligament tenderness	Inability to bear weight
Localized lateral swelling	Antalgic gait	Gait modification
Antalgic gait	Adduction/abduction movements are painful	Swelling localized and proximal to the ankle joint
Joint laxity		Inability to "push off"
Heard a "pop" or "snap"		Pain radiating proximally from the ankle joint

References

1. Clifton D, Phan K, Zimmerman E. Utilizing Ottawa ankle rules to enhance clinical decision making. *NATA News*. 2013;25:42-43.
2. Boytim M, Fischer D, Neumann L. Syndesmotic ankle sprains. *Am J Sports Med*. 1991;19:294-298.
3. Amendola A, Williams G, Foster D. Evidence-based approach to treatment of acute traumatic syndesmosis (high ankle) sprains. *Sports Med Arthroscopy Rev*. 2006;14:232-236.
4. Hopkinson W, St Pierre P, Ryan J, Wheeler J. Syndesmosis sprains of the ankle. *Foot Ankle*. 1990;10:325-330.
5. Nussbaum E, Hosea T, Sieler S, Incremona B, Kessler D. Prospective evaluation of syndesmotic ankle sprains without diastasis. *Am J Sports Med*. 2001;29:31-35.

WHAT ARE THE MOST USEFUL CLINICAL TESTS TO ACCURATELY DIAGNOSE SYNDESMOTIC AND MEDIAL ANKLE SPRAINS?

Eric Nussbaum, MEd, ATC, LAT and
James C. Sullivan, DPM, ATC, FACFAS

Clinical Tests for Syndesmotic Ankle Sprains

Clinical evaluation of the ankle syndesmosis includes not just radiographic evaluation and taking a good history but also several dynamic tests used to assess the stability of the joint. None of these tests is 100% predictive or specific enough to note specific laxity or to identify the degree of ligament injury but, when positive, are often indicative of syndesmotic injury. Clinicians should have a high level of suspicion for patients who exhibit functional disability, tenderness, distinctive swelling above the classic ankle joint, and extreme pain. A tape measure may also be used to note increased volume at the syndesmosis (Figure 12-1).

Clinical examination should start with a thorough history to try to determine the mechanism and prior history of injury. Reports of an injury mechanism involving rotation coupled with pain at extreme ranges of dorsiflexion or plantar flexion should be met with a high level of suspicion of a syndesmotic sprain.

McKeon PO, Wikstrom EA, eds. *Quick Questions in
Ankle Sprains: Expert Advice in Sports Medicine* (pp 63-67).
© 2015 SLACK Incorporated.

Figure 12-1. Increased volume/size associated with syndesmotic injury.

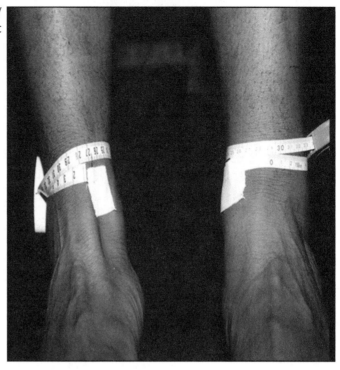

PALPATION

Tenderness noted with palpation of the anterior and/or posterior inferior tibio-fibular ligaments is clinically significant. The most frequently injured ligament of the syndesmsosis is the anterior inferior tibiofibular ligament, which runs diagonally from the distal lateral tibia to the medial side of the fibula. The ligament is easy to palpate and when tender should increase suspicion of a syndesmotic sprain.[5,6] The most common remark of a patient who presents with a syndesmotic sprain is that he or she has trouble "pushing off." The single-leg hop test (SLHT) can be used to identify individuals who are unable to push off.

SINGLE-LEG HOP TEST

Before asking an athlete to do a hop test, the clinician should ask him or her to bear weight with weight shifts and then transition to double toe raises. The patient is asked to perform a single-leg hop from his or her toes 5 times in a row. If the patient cannot hop, syndesmotic injury should be considered.[5] A key to doing the SLHT is to instruct the athlete to hop from his or her toes without allowing the heel to touch the ground. Some patients will be able to hop flatfooted but will be unable to do so while keeping their heels off the ground. This is a great test to do on the sidelines as a quick assessment for the functional ability of a person suspected of having a syndesmotic sprain. As well, this test can be used prior to starting more functional skills in an athlete's rehabilitation progression and return-to-play activity. In a comparative study the SLHT had the highest sensitivity.[6]

The most common mechanism of injury for a syndesmotic ankle sprain is combined dorsiflexion, external rotation, and hyperpronation. Therefore, clinical tests that stress these joint movements and replicate the mechanism of injury may help to identify the injury.

MODIFIED KLEIGER TEST (EXTERNAL ROTATION; HYPERPRONATION)

A classic Kleiger test is described as externally rotating the foot while stabilizing the lower leg. If this creates pain, it is considered a positive result. It is noted to have the highest degree of intertester reliability and the lowest rate of false-positive results when compared with other syndesmotic tests.[1]

A modified Kleiger test incorporates dorsiflexion of the foot and external rotation in an attempt to improve reliability. The test has a high level of sensitivity.[6] The Kleiger test is unable to determine joint laxity; rather, the examiner is looking for the reproduction of pain, which may be indicative of injury.

SQUEEZE TEST

First described by Bilik, this test is completed by squeezing the tibia and fibula together at midcalf and looking for pain at the ankle joint. A positive test is indicated with ankle pain when the lower leg bones are compressed. Biomechanical analysis confirmed that the test causes separation at the distal tibiofibular joint. It is thought to increase tension in the remaining ankle syndesmosis ligament fibers, resulting in pain at the ankle.[6] When compared with other syndesmotic tests, this test has been shown to have poor interexaminer reliability,[1,3] but when positive, the test has been shown to correlate with a longer return to participation.[5]

Since syndesmotic injury can result in increased joint space, additional tests to consider for evaluation of the syndesmosis use tape or the examiner's hands to compress the malleoli, restoring joint stability, while the patient moves through a range of motion. Clinical significance is noted when this range-of-motion increases. Examples of tests that incorporate compression and movement are the dorsiflexion lunge with compression test, the tape test,[2] and the malleolar compression/rebound test.[4]

Clinical Tests for Medial Ankle Sprains

Medial ankle injury is the least common injury of the ankle joint, accounting for only 5% to 10% of ankle sprains, but it can have a significant impact on ankle function. Evaluations of the medial ankle joint should assess the deltoid ligament, but also evaluate the major structures that cross the joint on the medial side, which may contribute to pain. Examiners should be cognizant that the deltoid ligament can be injured in a mechanism similar to that which may create injury to the ankle syndesmosis (hyperpronation). Notation of pain over the medial ankle with any of the above-mentioned tests for syndesmotic ankle sprains should be considered suspicious.

Tests for the medial ankle should include the following:

- Focal palpation of the deltoid ligament, medial tendons, tarsal tunnel, distal tibia, and fibula; tenderness should be noted.

- The Cotton test, which involves stabilizing the lower leg, grasping the calcaneous, and rocking it medially/laterally looking for painful motion and joint laxity, may help to identify deltoid injury. Severe medial ankle sprains can produce significant joint instability, which should be apparent when using the Cotton test.

- The talar tilt test, though classically used to access the lateral ankle, may be provocative and cause medial pain.

Because of the strength and thickness of the ligament and the position of the distal fibula below the tibiotalar joint, frank, occult, and avulsion fracture of the distal fibula and tibia should always be considered with deltoid injury. Examiners should follow Ottawa ankle rules and always rule out a fracture with medial-sided injury.

The musculotendenous junction of the posterior tibial tendon, flexor halluces, and the flexor digitorum tendon can be injured when an athlete has rotational and dorsiflexion components, which may create pathology. Longitudinal split tears of the medial tendons are not uncommon in the athletic population and are often missed clinically. Palpation, manual muscle testing, and functional evaluations can help to identify subtle pathology to the medial tendons. Further imaging may be needed to clarify the extent of injury.

Equally important to consider with the suspicion of a medial ankle sprain is the neurovascular structures within the tarsal tunnel. Although traction and direct trauma injuries to the tibial nerve have a more distinctive clinical presentation, this important area of the medial ankle should always be evaluated for injury.

Hyperdorsiflexion, external rotation, and/or hyperpronation may injure the ankle syndesmosis and the structures of the medial ankle. It is therefore important to thoroughly evaluate these structures for injury when history and clinical findings raise suspicion.

References

1. Alonso A. Clinical tests for ankle syndesmosis injury: reliability and predication of return to function. *J Orthop Sports Phys Ther.* 1998;27:276-284.
2. Amendola A. Evidence-based approach to treatment of acute traumatic syndesmosis sprains. *Sports Med Arthrosc.* 2006;14:232-236.
3. Beumer A. Clinical diagnosis of syndesmotic ankle instability: evaluation of stress tests behind the curtains. *Acta Orthop Scand.* 2002;73:667-669.
4. Mulligan EP. Evaluation and management of ankle syndesmosis injuries. *Phys Ther Sport.* 2011;12:57-69.
5. Nussbaum E. Prospective evaluation of syndesmotic ankle sprains without diastasis. *Am J Sport Med.* 2001;29:31-35.
6. Sman A. Diagnostic accuracy of clinical tests for diagnosis of ankle syndesmosis injury: a systematic review. *BJSM Online.* 2013;47:620-628.

WHAT ARE THE MOST USEFUL CLINICAL TESTS FOR ACCURATELY DIAGNOSING ACUTE LATERAL ANKLE SPRAINS?

Cathleen N. Brown, PhD, ATC;
Adam B. Rosen, PhD, ATC; and Jupil Ko, MS, ATC

Lateral ankle sprains are a common injury, and inversion and plantar flexion is the typical mechanism. A lateral ankle sprain most often results in either isolated or combined injuries of the anterior talofibular ligament (ATFL) or the calcaneofibular ligament (CFL).[1] The ATFL prevents anterior translation of the talus on the tibia, and the CFL prevents inversion. Acute lateral ankle sprains may prohibit people from participating in physical and daily living activities because of pain and disability. It is important to appropriately identify these injuries to access appropriate care and treatment to ensure recovery.

Clinical tests are commonly applied during physical examination of acute lateral ankle sprains to determine if the ATFL, CFL, or both are injured and how severely,[2] usually as confirmatory tests at the end of the evaluation.[3] Such tests are advantageous, because they are inexpensive, quick to administer, and typically accessible in clinical and field settings for determining referral, removal, or return to play.[1,4] Ideally, clinical tests should demonstrate strong evidence-based foundations including good interrater and intrarater reliability, sensitivity, specificity, and positive and negative likelihood ratios. However, not all those factors are evident

McKeon PO, Wikstrom EA, eds. *Quick Questions in Ankle Sprains: Expert Advice in Sports Medicine* (pp 69-74).
© 2015 SLACK Incorporated.

with tests for lateral ankle sprains. The purpose of this chapter is to present evidence for usefulness and recommendations for several clinical tests for a lateral ankle sprain.

Clinical Tests

ANTERIOR DRAWER

In the commonly used anterior drawer test, the examiner uses one hand to stabilize the tibia distally and uses the other to pull the foot anteriorly at the calcaneus to check the integrity of the ATFL.[5] A positive anterior drawer test is likely to indicate acute ATFL injury due to lateral ankle sprain, but a negative test does not necessarily rule out injury (Table 13-1).[3] In cadaver ankles with sectioned ligaments, the anterior drawer test was not sensitive enough to determine the degree of injury due to variability between the examiners and cadavers, and a neutral ankle position was not necessarily better than plantar flexion for test position.[2] Other cadaver studies with sectioned ligaments found a fair-to-good correlation between the rater's "appreciation" of instability and directly measured anatomic motion, although these correlations were not always statistically significant.[1,5] With a cut point of 3 mm or more of translation for a positive test, the sensitivity was good and the specificity was moderate.[1] When the cut point increased to ≥ 4 mm, sensitivity was excellent and specificity was good.[5] Using cadavers with completely sectioned ligaments, blinded raters' intrarater reliability was excellent, but interrater reliability was only moderate.[5] However, when patients with variable ankle sprain history were tested, experienced raters' interrater reliability was poor, as was the overall interrater reliability for both experienced and novice raters (see Table 13-1).[4]

TALAR TILT

Another common test is the talar tilt, in which the examiner stabilizes the distal tibia with one hand while inverting the calcaneus with the other, attempting to judge laxity at the talocrural joint and CFL. A positive talar tilt test provides moderate sensitivity and good specificity and predicts small but possibly important shifts in the likelihood of ligamentous damage.[3] A cadaveric study with sectioned ligaments reported significant increases in degree of talar tilt in neutral and 20 degrees of plantar flexion when the test was applied between the ATFL and CFL sections but not between intact ligaments and the initial ATFL sectioning.[2] Thus, the talar tilt test seems most appropriate for CFL or combined ATFL/CFL injury, not isolated ATFL injury. However, the degree of ankle ligament injury could not be accurately determined because of variability between the examiners

Table 13-1

Diagnostic Accuracy of Selected Clinical Tests for Lateral Ankle Sprain

Test	Sensitivity[4]	Specificity	Positive Likelihood Ratio	Negative Likelihood Ratio	Interrater Reliability	Intrarater Reliability
Anterior drawer	0.58[3] ≥3-mm cut point 0.75[1] ≥4-mm cut point 1.00[5]	1.00[3] ≥3-mm cut point 0.50[1] ≥4-mm cut point 0.67[5]	Undefined[3]	0.42[3]	0.06 to 0.16[4] 0.52[5]	0.94[5]
Talar tilt	0.50[3]	0.88[3]	4.0[3]	0.57[3]	0.29 to 0.33[4]	
Anterolateral drawer	≥3-mm cut point 1.00[1] ≥4-mm cut point 1.00[5]	≥3-mm cut point 1.00[1] ≥4-mm cut point 0.67[5]			0.52[5]	0.80[5]
Medial subtalar glide	0.58[3]	0.88[3]	4.67[3]	0.48[3]		

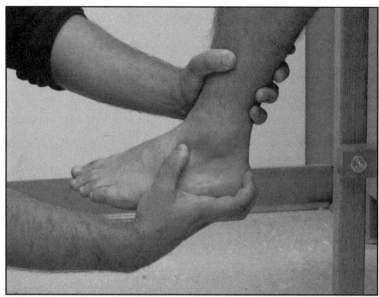

Figure 13-1. Anterolateral drawer test. The distal tibia is fixed with one hand above the malleoli while the other hand grasps the posterior heel using the index and middle fingers. The thumb is placed on the articulation of the lateral talus and anterior aspect of the distal fibula. The ankle is placed in 10 to 15 degrees of plantar flexion while the heel is pushed anteriorly, allowing the talus to internally rotate.

and cadavers.[2] Using patients with variable ankle sprain histories, the experienced raters' interrater reliability was poor, as was the overall interrater reliability for both experienced and novice raters for both patient positions (see Table 13-1).[4]

OTHER CLINICAL TESTS

There is some evidence to support other less common or newer clinical tests to evaluate acute lateral ankle sprains. In the anterolateral drawer test (Figure 13-1), the examiner uses one hand's thumb, web space, and index finger to stabilize the leg just above the malleoli. The other hand's palm supports the sole and places the ankle in 10 to 15 degrees of plantar flexion, while the index and other fingers stabilize the posterior heel and apply the anterior force. The thumb is placed 1 cm proximal to the tip of the lateral malleolus, longitudinally on the lateral joint line along the lateral aspect of the anterior talar dome. When the anterior force is applied to the calcaneus, the foot is allowed to internally rotate and the thumb palpates translation and any step-off.[1] This test displayed a good-to-excellent, and statistically significant, correlation between a rater's "appreciation" of instability and direct anatomic measures of ligament laxity on cadavers after progressive ligament sectioning.[1,5] The results may be different in vivo and with a different number of days after injury. When 3 mm or more of translation was used as a cut point, sensitivity and specificity were excellent with one experienced rater.[1] When 4 mm or more was used, sensitivity was excellent and specificity was good with a variety of experienced and inexperienced raters.[5] Intrarater reliability was good and inter-rater reliability was moderate (see Table 13-1).[5]

The medial subtalar glide requires the examiner to stabilize the talus in neutral with one hand while using the other to glide the calcaneus medially on the fixed talus and assess the amount of translation, possibly incorporating the cervical and interosseous ligaments, CFL, and lateral talocalcaneal and fibulotalocalcaneal ligaments. The sensitivity was moderate, with good-to-excellent specificity, and small but possibly important shifts in probability if the test was positive.[3] There is little information about the role of the subtalar joint in lateral ankle sprains, and no other commonly used tests target this joint. A positive test result seems to be a good indicator that subtalar laxity may be present after ankle sprain, but it likely needs to be used in addition to the tests above, because it evaluates different structures.

Conclusion

In patients, the anterior drawer, talar tilt, and medial subtalar glide tests have moderate-to-good sensitivity and good-to-excellent specificity individually, but may overestimate clinicians' ability to use them to diagnose a lateral ankle sprain.[3] The anterior drawer test has had moderate usefulness in cadavers, while the antero-lateral drawer test has appeared a bit more useful.[1] Additionally, reliability within and between clinicians is still poor, especially across a range of patient populations.[4] Using grading scales with only a few levels may improve the reliability of manual testing.[4] Some tests, such as the anterolateral drawer test, may be more useful to novice clinicians than established tests such as the anterior drawer test.[5]

Following an ankle sprain, changes in degree of laxity are small but may be relevant despite a lack of statistically significant changes.[4] Clinicians frequently use these tests to grade ankle sprains, but the manual tests may be unreliable and are not highly correlated to self-reported function or degree of ligamentous damage.[2,4] Our current tests for evaluating the severity of lateral ankle sprains may not be very good and may cause us to underestimate the actual damage from the injury, which could be contributing to the high rate of recurrence. Some newer or modified tests may be better options for clinical assessment of acute lateral ankle sprains.[5] Whichever manual tests are chosen, clinicians should standardize their approach and interpret their results with caution.

References

1. Phisitkul P, Chaichankul C, Sripongsai R, et al. Accuracy of anterolateral drawer test in lateral ankle instability: a cadaveric study. *Foot Ankle Int.* 2009;30:690-695.
2. Fujii T, Luo ZP, Kitaoka HB, An KN. The manual stress test may not be sufficient to differentiate ankle ligament injuries. *Clin Biomech.* 2000;15:619-623.
3. Schwieterman B, Haas D, Columber K, Knupp D, Cook C. Diagnostic accuracy of physical examination tests of the ankle/foot complex: a systematic review. *Int J Sports Phys Ther.* 2013;8:416-426.
4. Wilkin EJ, Hunt A, Nightingale EJ, et al. Manual testing for ankle instability. *Man Ther.* 2012;17:593-596.
5. Vaseenon T, Gao Y, Phisitkul P. Comparison of two manual tests for ankle laxity due to rupture of the lateral ankle ligaments. *Iowa Orthop J.* 2012;32:9-16.

How Well Do the Ottawa Ankle and Foot Rules Help to Accurately Rule Out Ankle Fracture?

Jeffrey D. Tiemstra, MD, FAAFP

Lateral ankle sprains are a very common injury, with an annual incidence of 2 per 1000 person-years in the general population, and more than 7 per 1000 person-years in teenagers aged 15 to 19 years.[1] Most of these patients have soft-tissue injuries, with only a small percentage experiencing a fracture. The Ottawa ankle and foot rules were developed to reduce the number of radiographs required by identifying specific physical examination findings that could reliably exclude the possibility of a fracture.

Lateral ankle sprains occur when the foot is "rolled," or inverted, resulting in the patient's body weight coming down on the lateral aspect of the foot and ankle. The 2 ligaments preventing this motion are the anterior talofibular ligament and the calcaneofibular ligament. In a lateral sprain, these ligaments are stretched or torn, resulting in pain, swelling, and bruising on both sides of the lateral malleolus (the distal end of the fibula). Because of the effects of gravity, within a few hours swelling and bruising may spread over the entire lateral aspect of the ankle and foot.

McKeon PO, Wikstrom EA, eds. *Quick Questions in Ankle Sprains: Expert Advice in Sports Medicine* (pp 75-78).

There are 4 types of bony injuries that can occur with a lateral ankle sprain.

1. In some cases, instead of the lateral ligaments themselves tearing, they will tear off the distal tip of the lateral malleolus. This is referred to as an avulsion fracture, and it will appear on radiographs as a small chip of bone torn away from the fibula and separated by a few millimeters.

2. The second type of bony injury involves the fifth metatarsal. The proximal end of the fifth metatarsal protrudes slightly outward. (It can be easily palpated along the lateral aspect of the foot.) With the foot inverted in a roll, the patient's body weight is directly over the proximal fifth metatarsal, in some cases resulting in a fracture.

3. The navicular bone, one of the small bones of the proximal midfoot (medial to top center of the foot just distal to the ankle joint), will sometimes partially dislocate in a lateral ankle sprain, especially if there is a rotation of the foot in addition to inversion.

4. The medial malleolus may be fractured by the force of the foot inverting into it.

Of patients seen in the emergency department with a lateral ankle sprain, about 10% to 20% will have an associated fracture. Since many patients with ankle sprains are either seen in an office setting or do not seek any medical care, the overall incidence of fractures associated with lateral ankle sprains is probably lower than 10%.

Researchers at the University of Ottawa developed a set of clinical guidelines to rule out the possibility of fracture and therefore avoid the need for radiographs in the 90% of patients who do not have a fracture. The first rule requires the patient to be able to bear weight for 4 steps both immediately after the injury and at the time of the examination. The next 4 rules require the absence of tenderness to palpation over the 4 bony areas of potential fracture/dislocation: the lateral malleolus, the proximal fifth metatarsal, the midfoot zone, and the medial malleolus. If the patient has tenderness over any of these bony areas, or cannot bear weight for 4 steps, then appropriate ankle and/or foot radiographs are needed. When palpating the foot, care must be taken to avoid palpating areas of soft-tissue injury, specifically the lateral ligaments of the ankle. When palpating the lateral malleolus, the examiner should use the fingertips only to palpate the posterior edge of the bone, avoiding the adjacent lateral ligaments as much as possible. Table 14-1 summarizes these rules.

The Ottawa ankle and foot rules were originally published in 1993.[2] Since then, there have been more than 100 published studies assessing and validating them. In 2003, a meta-analysis of 27 of the highest-quality studies was published, and it included 15,881 patients.[3] This study reported an overall sensitivity of 99.7% for the rules' ability to rule out a fracture when all 5 criteria are met. The rules have

Table 14-1
The Ottawa Ankle and Foot Rules

Rule	Radiographs Needed if Failed
Bear weight for 4 steps immediately after injury and during examination?	Ankle and/or foot
Tenderness along posterior edge of lateral malleolus?	Ankle
Tenderness along posterior edge of medial malleolus?	Ankle
Tenderness over proximal fifth metatarsal?	Foot
Tenderness over midfoot, navicular bone?	Foot

been tested in children and found to be equally effective. A 2009 meta-analysis of 12 studies in children as young as 5 years, with 3135 patients, reported an overall sensitivity of 98.5% for excluding a fracture.[4] In that analysis, only 10 of 671 fractures were missed, and 4 of the 10 were deemed clinically insignificant.

It is important to remember that the Ottawa rules are not very accurate at diagnosing a fracture. Studies have found low and quite variable rates of fractures in patients who fail one or more of the rules. Overall, patients who fail one or more of the Ottawa rules have only a 20% to 50% risk of having a fracture. Keep in mind that the purpose of the rules is not to diagnose a fracture but to reliably exclude the possibility of a fracture and thus avoid an unnecessary radiograph. Studies have consistently found that application of the Ottawa ankles rules can reduce the number of radiographs by 30% to 40%.

Conclusion

Application of the Ottawa ankle and foot rules can eliminate one-third of the radiographs taken for sprained ankles. Patients who pass all 5 rules can be reassured that they have less than a 1% chance of a fracture. Patients who fail one or more rules have a 20% to 50% risk of a fracture and should have appropriate ankle and foot radiographs.

References

1. Waterman BR, Owens BD, Davey S, Zacchilli MA, Belmont PJ Jr. The epidemiology of ankle sprains in the United States. *J Bone Joint Surg Am*. 2010;92:2279-2284.
2. Stiell IG, Greenberg GH, McKnight RD, et al. Decision rules for the use of radiography in acute ankle injuries. Refinement and prospective validation. *JAMA*. 1993;269(9):1127-1132.
3. Bachmann LM, Kolb E, Koller MT, Steurer J, ter Riet G. Accuracy of Ottawa ankle rules to exclude fractures of the ankle and mid-foot: systematic review. *BMJ*. 2003;326:417.
4. Dowling S, Spooner CH, Liang Y, et al. Accuracy of Ottawa ankle rules to exclude fractures of the ankle and midfoot in children: a meta-analysis. *Acad Emerg Med*. 2009;16:277-287.

WHAT ARE THE CONCOMITANT INJURIES THAT OCCUR WITH A LATERAL ANKLE SPRAIN?

J. Ty Hopkins, PhD, ATC, FNATA, FACSM

The ankle is a joint complex with multiple articulations, multiple degrees of freedom, and multiple axes of rotation. With this in mind, and given the high loads that pass through the joint, it is no surprise that the ankle is often injured. Inversion ankle sprains are extremely common, and while the injury often seems simple, there are a number of associated conditions that should be considered. This chapter explores conditions that can accompany or naturally follow an inversion ankle sprain. These conditions fall into 1 of 3 categories: (1) conditions associated with the acute injury mechanism, (2) conditions associated with adaptations in the subacute phases following injury, and (3) conditions associated with chronic adaptations following injury.

Conditions Associated With Acute Inversion Ankle Sprain Mechanisms

Most ankle injuries occur when the foot is forced into inversion or supination. When the talus is forced medially (often in conjunction with internal rotation) in the mortise, a number of structures outside of the lateral ankle ligaments are exposed to forces that can cause injury. Each of these injuries should be ruled out after a lateral ankle sprain.

McKeon PO, Wikstrom EA, eds. *Quick Questions in Ankle Sprains: Expert Advice in Sports Medicine* (pp 79-82). © 2015 SLACK Incorporated.

Let us consider how the bones and associated articular cartilage might be affected by this mechanism. When the talus is forced medially, it can contact the medial malleolus, resulting in a distal tibial fracture. This same mechanism, along with internal rotation, can cause significant impact to the talus as the edge rubs against the distal tibia, causing a contusion. The contusion can lead to softening of the articular cartilage, possibly resulting in a talar dome articular cartilage lesion. Depending on the size of the lesion, the articular cartilage may have a difficult time healing. On the lateral side, the distal fibular malleolus may be avulsed from the pull of the calcaneofibular ligament during forced inversion, and the base of the fifth metatarsal is often avulsed from a combination of the tension generated by inversion and by the contraction of the peroneus brevis.

Other conditions to consider with the described mechanism include injuries to the peroneal musculotendinous unit, anterior tibiofibular ligaments, the syndesmosis, and the lateral retinaculum. While these conditions may be more common with forced dorsiflexion and/or external rotation, any traumatic ankle sprain could result in forcing the distal tibia and fibula apart, damaging the high ligaments and syndesmosis. The lateral retinaculum could be exposed on forced inversion while the evertors contract, causing rupture of the retinaculum. The result would be a chronically subluxing peroneal tendon during this type of movement.

Pain, swelling, instability, and immobility often accompany each of these conditions, making them difficult to distinguish from an ankle sprain. Chondral injury often results in constant deep aching in addition to other signs and symptoms. Appropriate diagnostics, including the Ottawa ankle rules,[1] should be included in the evaluation process to ensure the correct course of care and treatment.

Conditions Associated With the Subacute Period After an Ankle Sprain

Due to the mechanism described above and short-term adaptations during the healing process (ie, scar tissue formation, adaptive shortening of tissues, etc), several conditions may manifest themselves in the weeks following injury. Clinicians should pay attention to these conditions during the rehabilitation process. Perhaps more common is the situation in which a patient or athlete presents weeks after injury and no formal treatment or rehabilitation has taken place.

Sinus tarsi syndrome is a condition that occurs secondary to acute ankle sprain(s). It is characterized by persistent anterolateral pain, often due to subtalar joint instability, resulting in excessive pronation and supination movements. These excessive movements cause additional stress on the capsule and ligaments in the sinus tarsi space, resulting in chronic inflammation and fibrosis.[2]

Impingement syndrome of the ankle is a condition characterized by chronic pain, and while somewhat rare, the most common patient population is 15- to 40-year-old athletes. Impingement syndrome is more specifically characterized as anterolateral, anterior, anteromedial, and posterior impingement. The first 3 are most often associated with inversion ankle sprains or other traumatic injury, while posterior impingement is associated with traumatic fractures or forced plantar flexion (ballet dancers, soccer players, etc). Impingement following injury or repeated injury is created by thickening of the capsule or capsular ligaments, synovitis, and/or osseous spurs; this creates a narrowing in the talocrural joint, which restricts motion and causes chronic pain. Pain is aggravated by forced movement in the direction of the impingement. Diagnosis should be confirmed radiographically.[3]

Positional faults of the talus and/or fibula can occur in conjunction with or secondary to ankle sprains. Several researchers and clinicians have hypothesized that an inversion injury results in an anterior shift of the fibula and/or the talus, resulting in less damage to the ligament but placing the bone in poor alignment with adjacent joint structures.[4] This poor position, or fault, results in pain from increased pressure or tension on joint structures and ultimately adaptive changes to the tissues involved. The result is poor arthrokinematics, resulting in limited osteokinematic movement, namely dorsiflexion. Limited dorsiflexion range of motion could result in increased ankle injury risk.

Conditions Associated With
Chronic Adaptations After an Ankle Sprain

Chronic adaptations to an ankle sprain can depend on many factors following injury. Some of these factors include how the acute injury is managed, the movement strategies that are adopted by the patient after injury, adaptive changes to tissues, damage to articular cartilage and subchondral bone, and the activity level of the patient or athlete. Depending on these and other factors, the original ankle sprain could balloon into something more consequential.

Chronic ankle instability (CAI) has been discussed in previous questions, and we do not discuss it in depth here. However, it is worth mentioning that CAI can be affected by each of the conditions that are discussed in this chapter. Additionally, sensorimotor alterations can play a large role in perpetuating the chronic nature of ankle instability.[5] While CAI is a complicated phenomenon that is still not well understood, the factors that are thought to contribute to this condition should be identified in an effort to reduce the risk of reinjury.

Some would argue that the ultimate risk of multiple ankle injuries and many of the conditions discussed in this chapter is that of degenerative disease of the articular cartilage and underlying bone. Premature ankle osteoarthritis is a condition that is highly related to multiple ankle injuries and instability. Currently, there are limited treatment options for ankle osteoarthritis, and as clinicians, we should be tireless in our efforts to prevent this condition. This means that we should work to prevent ankle injury, and when an ankle sprain does occur, we should be careful to return an athlete to competition only when he or she is ready.

Ankle injury will continue to be a common athletic injury. Clinicians should be familiar with the concomitant injuries that can occur and possible consequences of each of them. By identifying and treating these conditions, we can positively influence the long-term health of the ankle and the patient.

References

1. Stiell I. Ottawa ankle rules. *Can Fam Physician.* 1996;42:478-480.
2. Pisani G, Pisani PC, Parino E. Sinus tarsi syndrome and subtalar joint instability. *Clin Podiatr Med Surg.* 2005;22:63-77.
3. Robinson P, White LM, Salonen D, Ogilvie-Harris D. Anteromedial impingement of the ankle: using MR arthrography to assess the anteromedial recess. *Am J Roentgenol.* 2002;178:601-604.
4. Vicenzino B, Branjerdporn M, Teys P, Jordan K. Initial changes in posterior talar glide and dorsiflexion of the ankle after mobilization with movement in individuals with recurrent ankle sprain. *J Orthop Sports Phys Ther.* 2006;36:464-471.
5. Hertel J. Sensorimotor deficits with ankle sprains and chronic ankle instability. *Clin Sports Med.* 2008;27:353-370.

WHAT CRITERIA SHOULD BE USED TO DIAGNOSE A PATIENT WITH CHRONIC ANKLE INSTABILITY?

Eamonn Delahunt, PhD, BSc (Physiotherapy), SMISCP;
Brian Caulfield, PhD, M MedSc, B Physio, MISCP; and
Cailbhe Doherty, BSc (Physiotherapy)

Lateral ankle sprain has been shown to represent a significant injury risk in a variety of activity types and is one of the most frequently incurred lower-limb musculoskeletal injuries by athletes.[1] Of particular concern to clinicians is the high reported incidence of residual symptoms that may manifest after a first-time lateral ankle sprain. *Chronic ankle instability* is the most commonly used term in the scientific literature to describe these residual symptoms. Chronic ankle instability has been defined as "an encompassing term used to classify a subject with both mechanical and functional instability of the ankle joint," whereby residual symptoms, including episodes of the ankle joint "giving way," subjective feelings of ankle joint instability, and recurrent sprain, are present for a minimum of 1 year after an initial lateral ankle joint sprain.[2] The subjective feeling of ankle instability commonly reported by patients, whereby activities of daily living and sports participation provoke a sensation that the ankle joint is unstable with an associated fear of sustaining an acute lateral ankle sprain, ultimately lends to the sense of giving way. Giving way is the characteristic most consistently reported by expert clinicians and researchers alike when defining chronic ankle instability.[2] Thus, giving way,

McKeon PO, Wikstrom EA, eds. *Quick Questions in*
Ankle Sprains: Expert Advice in Sports Medicine (pp 83-86).
© 2015 SLACK Incorporated.

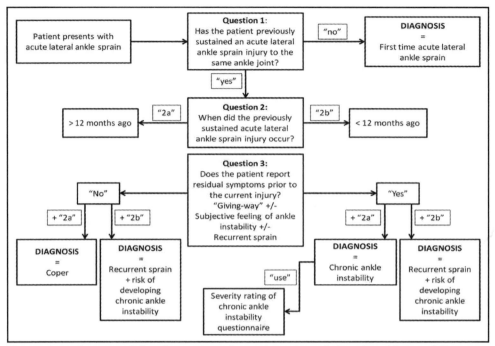

Figure 16-1. Framework for diagnosis and severity rating of chronic ankle instability.

defined as "the regular occurrence of uncontrolled and unpredictable episodes of excessive inversion of the rear foot (usually experienced during initial contact during walking or running), which do not result in an acute lateral ankle sprain," is the central characteristic residual symptom of chronic ankle instability, with recurrent ankle sprain being the primary manifestation of chronic ankle instability.[2] A patient can be defined as having recurrent ankle sprain if he or she has incurred a minimum of 2 acute lateral ankle sprains on the same lower limb.[2]

We present here a stepwise framework to aid clinicians in the diagnosis and severity rating of chronic ankle instability (Figure 16-1). This stepwise framework should be applied when a patient presents with an acute lateral ankle joint sprain.

Question 1: Has the patient previously sustained an acute lateral ankle sprain injury to the same ankle joint?

Answer "yes": Proceed with subjective questioning (proceed to Question 2).

Answer "no": Diagnosis can be considered a first-time acute lateral ankle sprain.

Question 2: When did the previously sustained acute lateral ankle sprain injury occur?

Answer "> 12 months ago" (a)

Answer "< 12 months ago" (b)

Question 3: Does the patient subjectively report the presence of giving-way episodes of the ankle joint with or without a subjective feeling of ankle instability with or without recurrent sprain prior to sustaining the current injury?

Answer "yes" + Answer 2(a): Diagnosis can be considered chronic ankle instability (proceed to use a questionnaire to determine severity of chronic ankle instability).

Answer "yes" + Answer 2(b): Diagnosis can be considered recurrent sprain plus risk of developing chronic ankle instability.

Answer "no" + Answer 2(a): Diagnosis can be considered "coper" with a new acute ankle joint sprain injury, whereby coper is described as the absence of chronic ankle instability associated residual symptoms following acute lateral ankle joint sprain.[3]

Answer "no" + Answer 2(b): Diagnosis can be considered recurrent sprain plus being at risk of developing chronic ankle instability.

Questionnaire: Use a condition-specific, self-reported questionnaire to determine the severity of chronic ankle instability. This may be used to guide rehabilitation practices, document recovery, and determine suitability of return to play when appropriate. If, from a subjective standpoint, a diagnosis of chronic ankle instability is determined, then it is advisable that clinicians use one of the following questionnaires to assess the severity of chronic ankle instability: the Cumberland ankle instability tool or the identification of functional ankle instability.[4,5]

Lateral ankle joint sprain is one of the most frequently encountered lower-limb musculoskeletal injuries in the clinical setting, and a large proportion of patients who incur a lateral ankle joint sprain will develop chronic ankle instability. As such, it is vital that clinicians be cognizant of the subjectively reported characteristic features of chronic ankle instability when considering such a diagnosis. These features include (1) an initial, significant lateral ankle joint sprain that occurred at least 1 year prior to the most recent consultation for lateral ankle joint sprain; (2) subsequent patient-reported episodes of ankle joint giving way; (3) patient-reported feelings of ankle joint instability; and (4) patient-reported recurrent ankle sprains. The presence of features 1 and 2 above are integral to the diagnosis of chronic ankle instability, and may be compounded by the presence of feature 3 and/or 4. An appropriate questionnaire can then be used to assess the severity of chronic ankle instability. Currently recommended questionnaires include the Cumberland ankle instability tool and the identification of functional ankle instability.[4,5]

References

1. Doherty C, Delahunt E, Caulfield B, et al. The incidence and prevalence of ankle sprain injury: a systematic review and meta-analysis of prospective epidemiological studies. *Sports Med*. 2014;44:123-140.
2. Delahunt E, Coughlan GF, Caulfield B, et al. Inclusion criteria when investigating insufficiencies in chronic ankle instability. *Med Sci Sports Exerc*. 2010;42:2106-2121.
3. Wikstrom EA, Brown CN. Minimum reporting standards for copers in chronic ankle instability research. *Sports Med*. 2014;44:251-268.
4. Hiller CE, Refshauge KM, Bundy AC, Herbert RD, Kilbreath SL. The Cumberland ankle instability tool: a report of validity and reliability testing. *Arch Phys Med Rehabil*. 2006;87:1235-1241.
5. Simon J, Donahue M, Docherty C. Development of the identification of functional ankle instability (IdFAI). *Foot Ankle Int*. 2012;33:755-763.

WHAT FUNCTIONAL TESTS BEST IDENTIFY FUNCTIONAL IMPAIRMENTS FOLLOWING A LATERAL ANKLE SPRAIN?

Carrie Docherty, PhD, ATC, FNATA

After a lateral ankle sprain, athletic trainers and other health care providers work to restore range of motion, strength, proprioception, and functional abilities. Functional abilities are particularly important when deciding if and when an athlete should return to sport participation. An array of functional performance tests for determining the extent of the functional deficits in people with a history of ankle sprain has been described in the literature. Generally, functional tests can be considered agility/speed or strength/power tests. Agility tests often incorporate a series of running or hopping tasks that require the participant to start, stop, and change directions. The main goal of these tests is to perform them as quickly as possible. These tests are often measured in terms of speed and/or number of errors that occurred during the test. Strength/power-related functional performance tests require more explosive activity. These tests are thought to assess muscle function and are measured by distance covered while completing the test. Some examples of functional performance tests that can be included in the different categories are listed in Table 17-1.

McKeon PO, Wikstrom EA, eds. *Quick Questions in*
Ankle Sprains: Expert Advice in Sports Medicine (pp 87-91).
© 2015 SLACK Incorporated.

Table 17-1

Examples of the Different Types of Functional Performance Tests Used to Assess Function of the Ankle

Functional Performance Test Category	Test Examples
Agility/speed test	Shuttle-run test
	Agility hop test
	Figure 8 hop test
	Single-limb hopping course
	Square-hop test
	Agility T-test
	Up-down-hop test
	Side-hop test
	6-meter crossover hop
Strength/power test	Single forward hop
	Triple forward hop
	Triple lateral hop
	Crossover hop
	Vertical jump

Regardless of how the test is classified, all functional performance tests require coordination of multiple joints and muscle groups as well as adequate range of motion, strength, balance, and neuromuscular control. The coordination of multiple systems to perform the task makes functional testing a critical component in return-to-play considerations. One criterion used by clinicians and researchers to determine functional readiness is by evaluating limb symmetry. To return to sport participation, the injured limb should be able to perform a test within 80% of the contralateral uninjured limb.[1] For this reason, functional tests that assess performance on only one limb at a time are most beneficial when determining functional abilities following an injury. Therefore, tests such as the shuttle-run test, the agility T-test, and the co-contraction test, which require the use of both limbs to complete the task, are not ideal.

Single-limb hopping tests have been found to be effective in identifying functional deficits following an ankle sprain. Specifically, the triple-forward-hop and the triple-lateral-hop tests are sensitive to change following a lateral ankle sprain.[1,2] In other words, these tests can quantify deficits in performance created by an acute injury or improvements in performance created through rehabilitation

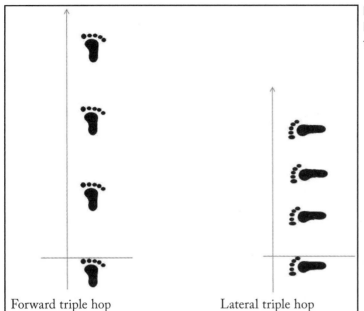

Figure 17-1. Forward-triple-hop and lateral-triple-hop tests.

Forward triple hop   Lateral triple hop

and/or healing of the injury. Both of these tests are performed on a single limb, and patients are asked to hop 3 times while covering as much distance as possible. The total distance covered by the 3 consecutive hops is recorded (Figure 17-1). Other speed/agility type-functional performance tests might also be useful in evaluating functional abilities following a lateral ankle sprain, but the studies in the published literature on these tests have primarily evaluated people with chronic ankle instability. There is a substantial amount of evidence reporting that people with chronic ankle instability have functional performance deficits while performing agility/speed-type tests; however, these tests have yet to be evaluated when determining deficits following an acute lateral ankle sprain. Examples of functional performance tests that have identified deficits in people with chronic ankle instability, and might be valuable in determining return-to-play criteria following a lateral ankle sprain, include the following: single-limb hopping test, figure 8 hopping test, side-hop test, square-hop test, and 6-meter crossover-hop test.[3,4]

Similar to what has been proposed in the literature for the postoperative anterior cruciate ligament, a battery of tests should be used when assessing functional performance for ankle sprains. This allows the clinician to use tests that evaluate both frontal and sagittal plane movement as well as both power and agility movements. Some functional tests, such as the single-limb hopping course (Figure 17-2) use sloped surfaces to further stress the ankle. This test used 8 squares and asks the participant to hop as quickly as possible through the course. Some of the squares slope laterally, while others have an incline or decline.[3,5] The different slopes stress different directional configurations that an athlete may encounter during sport

Figure 17-2. Single-limb hopping course.

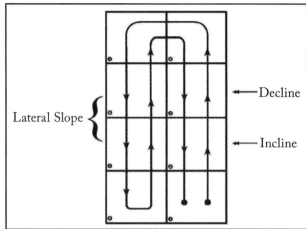

participation. The single-limb hopping course has been used to identify performance deficits in people with functional ankle instability. Another example that might be used in functional performance testing is asking the participant to perform a multiple-hop test in a particular pattern as quickly as possible. These tasks can be made more challenging by requiring the participant to balance in between jumps and/or by adding hurdles to a course, which requires them to maneuver a barrier. These functional performance tests stress the skeletal, muscular, and nervous systems of the body in a controlled environment to assist in determining if the participant should begin more strenuous activity. Another advantage to most functional performance tests is that they can be conducted with minimal to no equipment. The majority of these tests can be completed with a standard stopwatch and a measuring tape.

During the performance of any functional test, the clinician should not only rely on the time or distance outcome but also evaluate the quality of the movement, which will assist in determining if the participant is using any compensatory mechanisms to complete the test. When specifically evaluating someone with a previous ankle sprain, the participant may deviate from his or her normal movement patterns at the knee, hip, or core to compensate for deficits at the ankle. Finally, the clinician should also ask patients how they feel while performing the test. Some previous research on people with a history of an ankle sprain have determined that while actual performance of the injured limb might be similar to that of the uninjured limb, the patient still reports feelings of instability or chronic ankle dysfunction.[1] Therefore, we must be aware that after an ankle sprain, people have different amounts of residual systems. Caffrey et al[4] found that some participants with a history of a lateral ankle sprain reported perceived ankle instability that affected their performance during an array of functional performance tests, while others with similar histories of ankle injuries could perform the functional tasks without any deficiencies. The presence of perceived instability should be an indication that additional rehabilitation should be completed prior to returning the participant to sport or other high levels of physical activity. Some believe that inadequate rehabilitation and early return to sport performance may be major contributing factors in the high rate of ankle reinjury and chronic ankle instability.

Conclusion

Both the triple-forward-hop and triple-lateral-hop tests appear to be effective in detecting deficits in ankle function. However, limited evidence has been generated for other functional performance tests to determine if they may also be effective following an ankle sprain. Both the triple-forward-hop and triple-lateral-hop tests are measured in distance covered, so it would be interesting to evaluate how a more speed/agility-focused test would detect these functional deficits. Regardless of which tests are used, 2 or more tests should be used to determine functional ability in participants following a lateral ankle sprain.

References

1. Gerber JP, Williams GN, Scoville CR, Arciero RA, Taylor DC. Persistent disability associated with ankle sprains: a prospective examination of an athletic population. *Foot Ankle Int.* 1998;19:653-660.
2. Johnson MR, Stoneman PD. Comparison of a lateral hop test versus a forward hop test for functional evaluation of alateral ankle sprains. *J Foot Ankle Surg.* 2007;46:162-174.
3. Buchanan A, Docherty CL, Schrader J. Functional performance testing in participants with functional ankle instability and in a healthy control group. *J Athl Train.* 2008;43:342-346.
4. Caffrey E, Docherty CL, Schrader J, Klossner J. The ability of 4 single-limb hopping tests to detect functional performance deficits in individuals with functional ankle instability. *J Orthop Sports Phys Ther.* 2009;39:799-806.
5. Sekir U, Yildiz Y, Hazneci B, Ors F, Aydin T. Effect of isokinetic training on strength, functionality and proprioception in athletes with functional ankle instability. *Knee Surg Sports Traumatol.* 2007;15:654-664.

WHAT DIAGNOSTIC IMAGING TECHNIQUES ARE USED TO FURTHER EVALUATE SYNDESMOTIC, MEDIAL, AND LATERAL ANKLE SPRAINS?

Leah H. Portnow, MD; Joseph Surace, DO;
Tennyson Maliro, MD; and Javier Beltran, MD

Ankle sprains are stretching or tearing injuries of supporting ankle ligaments. These injuries occur in athletes and non-athletes by various ways but are often a result of abnormal motion and rotation. The best imaging technique for evaluating ligament injuries is magnetic resonance imaging (MRI). Images are obtained along an oblique axis in relation to the long axis of the metatarsals.[1] MRI resolves soft tissue structures such as ligaments more clearly. It provides multiplanar views: sagittal, lateral; coronal, front to back; and axial, head to toe. These various views enable full visualization of both the deep and superficial ligaments. The standard pulse MRI sequences include T1/fat-sensitive images, in which fat appears bright, and T2/fluid-sensitive images, in which fluid appears bright. The normal appearance of ligaments is thin and straight linear bands with black signal intensity on all sequences. Small, smooth gray lines can be seen within the medial collateral (deltoid) ligament, the posterior talofibular ligament of the lateral ligament complex, and the posterior syndesmotic ligament, but none should be as bright as fluid.[1]

Syndesmotic injuries are high ankle sprains. The components of the syndesmosis include the anterior and posterior tibiofibular ligaments and the interosseous ligament (Figure 18-1A). Sprains are often associated with ankle fractures. An

McKeon PO, Wikstrom EA, eds. *Quick Questions in Ankle Sprains: Expert Advice in Sports Medicine* (pp 93-96).

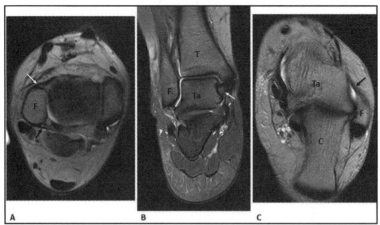

Figure 18-1. Normal syndesmotic, deltoid, and lateral ligaments. (A) Syndesmotic ligaments. An axial PD fat-saturated MR image of the distal tibia and fibula demonstrates normal syndesmotic ligaments with low signal, the anterior tibiofibular ligament (white arrow), and the posterior tibiofibular ligament (black arrow). (B) Deltoid ligaments. A PD fat-saturated coronal MR image demonstrates a normal deep deltoid ligament (white arrow) with its striated, low-intermediate signal-intensity fibers. (C) Lateral ligaments. An axial T1-weighted/fat-sensitive MR image of the distal fibula and talus demonstrates a normal anterior talofibular ligament with low signal (black arrow). T = tibia; F = fibula; Ta = talus; C = calcaneus.

accompanying medial ligament injury may be present. Some findings on radiographs that may hint to injury include the absence of the tibiofibular overlap, the overlap between the anterior tubercle of the tibia and medial border of the fibula 1 cm above the tibial plafond, and a greater than 6-mm tibiofibular clear space, the distance between the posteriolateral border of the tibia and the medial border of the fibula.[2] Widening of the tibiofibular clear space is evident in cases of complete disruption due to instability of the ankle mortise.[3] The Lauge-Hansen fracture classification is a method for categorizing ankle injury on the basis of mechanism of trauma, including foot position (supination or pronation) and direction of impact (abduction, adduction, and external rotation). In most studies, the Lauge-Hansen classification can detect syndesmotic ankle sprains in conjunction with fractures.[2] However, radiographs can commonly miss the less severe injury of partial tears in which only the anterior tibiofibular ligament is affected.[3] Studies show that the Lauge-Hansen system fails to detect anterior tibiofibular ligament tears, especially with supination-adduction injury, and posterior tibiofibular ligament injury in association with the anterior tibiofibular ligament.[2] Computed tomography (CT) can detect widening of the tibiofibular clear space better than radiographs and is more useful in uncovering avulsion fractures, which are associated with approximately 50% of syndesmotic ankle sprains.[3] MRI, in which injured ligaments are

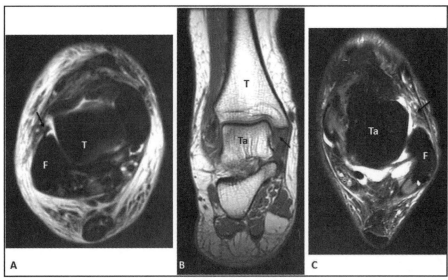

Figure 18-2. Ligament sprains. (A) Anterior syndesmotic ligament tear. An axial T2-weighted/fluid-sensitive fat-saturated MR image shows a completely torn anterior tibiofibular ligament (black arrow) with heterogeneous signal. (B) Deltoid ligament sprain. A T1-weighted/fat-sensitive coronal MR image demonstrates amorphous signal of the deep fibers of the deltoid ligament (black arrow) that indicates a sprain. (C) Lateral ligament tear. An axial T2-weighted/fluid-sensitive fat-saturated MR image shows a completely torn anterior talofibular ligament (white arrow) with heterogeneous signal. T = tibia; F = fibula; Ta = talus.

thick and show changes in signal intensity (Figure 18-2A), is still considered the gold standard.

The medial collateral ligament, or deltoid ligament, is composed of superficial and deep ligaments that attach the medial malleolus of the tibia to the tarsal bones of the foot. The superficial ligaments are the tibiocalcaneal, tibionavicular, and posterior superficial tibiotalar ligaments and the tibiospring ligament, which joins a portion of the spring ligament proper to stabilize the medial ankle. The deep layer consists of the anterior and posterior deep tibiotalar ligaments (Figure 18-1B). A sprain of the deltoid ligament is often due to various mechanisms, but especially with pronation and eversion.[4] However, clinical symptoms of medial ankle tenderness do not correlate with deltoid ligament injury.[4] Furthermore, ankle radiographs are not sensitive enough to detect this injury. A possible indication on radiographs of injury is widening greater than its normal 4 mm of the medial tibiotalar clear space, the space between the talus 5 mm below the articular surface, and the medial tibia.[4] The mortise view is the best way to see a widened medial tibiotalar clear space, but that finding is not an accurate predictor of deep ligament injury.[4] Fractures seen on radiographs that are classified as stable by the Lauge-Hansen system can be associated with a deep-ligament injury.[4] Therefore, MRI is the imaging modality of choice for accurate and early diagnosis. A grade 1 sprain, the most common type, is when the ligament is stretched and edematous. The normal striations of the deep ligaments are lost, and signal intensity is amorphous on fat-sensitive sequences (Figure 18-2B).[1] In partial tears (grade 2) and complete tears (grade 3), the deep ligaments are brighter and thicker on fluid-sensitive sequences.[1,4]

Lateral ligament sprains are the most common, accounting for about 85% of all injuries.[5] Its components include the anterior and posterior talofibular ligaments and the calcaneofibular ligament (Figure 18-1C). Usually, the anterior talofibular ligament is torn first, as it is the weakest, followed by the calcaneofibular and then the posterior talofibular ligament.[1] Again, we see the usefulness of MRI. Other imaging modalities are less specific. Stress view radiographs are difficult to obtain in acute injury secondary to pain, variability in normal angle of rotation to obtain the views, and the potential for worsening the injury.[5] Ultrasound depends on the expertise of the technician, and therefore sensitivity in detecting sprains varies, making the test unreliable.[5] Arthrography is not only similar in sensitivity to basic physical examination techniques that may be able to aid in diagnosis, but it is not recommended because it is invasive.[5] In MRI, a torn lateral ligament is clearly evident with changes in size and shape from the normal. It can become thinner or thicker, be irregular or wave-like, and change in signal intensity (Figure 18-2C).[1] MRI is typically obtained for competitive athletes when surgical repair may be required or to prevent chronic instability.

Conclusion

The diagnostic imaging techniques to best evaluate syndesmotic, medial, and lateral ankle sprains are fairly straightforward. Although radiographs via the Lauge-Hansen classification and CT may be beneficial in evaluating ankle sprain association with fractures, it is MRI that remains the gold standard. MRI has the best capability for determining torn ligaments with a variety of 3-dimensional reconstructions and is the most nonintrusive and specific technique.

References

1. Rosenberg ZS, Beltran J, Bencardino JT. From the RSNA refresher courses: MR imaging of the ankle and foot. *RadioGraphics*. 2000;20:S153-S179.
2. Hermans JJ, Wentink N, Beumer A, et al. Correlation between radiological assessment of acute ankle fractures and syndesmotic injury on MRI. *Skeletal Radiol*. 2012;41:787-801.
3. Molinari A, Stolley M, Amendola A. High ankle sprains (syndesmotic) in athletes: diagnostic challenges and review of the literature. *Iowa Orthop J*. 2009;29:130-138.
4. Chhabra A, Subhawong TK, Carrino JA. MR imaging of deltoid ligament pathologic findings and associated impingement syndromes. *RadioGraphics*. 2010;30:751-761.
5. Polzer H, Kanz KG, Prall WC, et al. Diagnosis and treatment of acute ankle injuries: development of an evidence-based algorithm. *Orthop Rev*. 2012;4(e5):22-32.

WHAT ARE IMPORTANT DIAGNOSTIC CONSIDERATIONS FOR THE PEDIATRIC ANKLE?

Claire E. Hiller, PhD, MAppSc, BAppSc (Physio) and
Joshua Burns, PhD, BAppSc (Pod)(Hons)

Pediatric ankle sprains occur more commonly than adult sprains. In fact, it has been estimated that there are more than 3 times as many ankle sprains in children and twice as many sprains in adolescents than in adults.[1] While diagnostic examination of the pediatric ankle is similar to that in adult populations, there are some specific considerations for both acute and chronic problems. In an acute ankle injury, the main consideration is the presence of a fracture, while in chronic problems the presence of other conditions should be suspected.

In the skeletally immature patient, it is important to detect the presence of any ankle fractures, as the development of asymmetrical or stunted bony growth may occur if correct treatment is not instituted. The lateral ankle ligaments in the skeletally immature patient attach to the tibia distal to the physeal line. When a rotational force is applied to the ankle during a low-velocity injury, the physeal area will often fail rather than the ligaments.[2] When the child has no closure of the physis, a Salter-Harris type I or II injury often occurs with a mechanism similar to that of lateral ankle sprain and is easily missed. Salter-Harris type I fractures cause a separation through the epiphyseal plate, whereas a type II fracture includes a fragment of metaphyseal bone (Figure 19-1). Salter-Harris type I injuries are often not discernable on plain radiographs, so careful palpation that elicits pain over the lateral

McKeon PO, Wikstrom EA, eds. *Quick Questions in
Ankle Sprains: Expert Advice in Sports Medicine* (pp 97-100).
© 2015 SLACK Incorporated.

Type	I	II	III	IV	V
Schematic	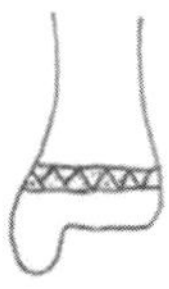	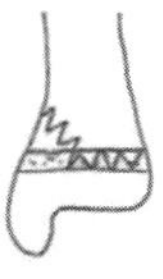	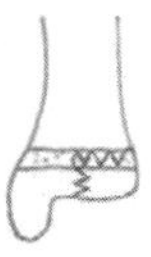	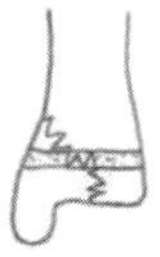	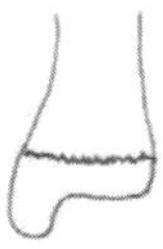
Fracture location	Along physis	Part of physis and metaphysis	Part of physis and epiphysis	Part of physis, epiphysis, and metaphysis	Crush of physis

Figure 19-1. Salter-Harris classification of fractures.

malleolus rather than the ligaments should raise suspicions. Isometric contraction of the lateral muscles around the joint will reproduce pain at the epiphyseal plate.

Salter-Harris type III fractures occur from the articular surface dorsally to the physis and then laterally along the physis. During adolescence, the physis first closes centrally and then medially and laterally. An external rotation force, similar to that causing a high ankle sprain in adults (syndesmosis), applied to the partially closed physis applies traction on the physis through the anterior talofibular ligament. This avulses a fragment of the lateral physis, which remains attached to the ligament. Both Tillaux (distal anterolateral quarter of the tibial physis) and triplane (3 tibial fragments) fractures can occur in the 18-month transitional period preceding physeal closure, which typically occurs at age 14 years in girls and age 16 years in boys.[3] These fractures are suspected with positive testing using the Ottowa ankle rules (refer to Question 14) and are usually clearly seen on plain radiographs.

Recently, a low-risk ankle rule has been developed to decrease the need to x-ray pediatric ankles.[2] A clinical examination that finds tenderness and swelling isolated to the distal fibula or adjacent lateral ligaments distal to the tibial anterior joint line does not require a radiograph (Figure 19-2). Low-risk ankle injuries include lateral ankle sprains, nondisplaced Salter-Harris type I and II fractures of the distal fibula, and avulsion fractures of the distal fibula or lateral talus.

Children presenting with chronic problems following an ankle injury, such as recurrent ankle sprains or ongoing pain, should be assessed for the presence of tarsal coalition, osteochondral talar dome lesion, or a neuromuscular disorder (eg, Charcot-Marie-Tooth [CMT] disease). All of these problems are described later.

A tarsal coalition may present in early adolescence following an ankle sprain. A coalition is the joining of 2 tarsal bones by a bony, cartilaginous, or fibrous union and occurs 3 times more commonly in boys than in girls. Common coalitions at the ankle that present as the coalition begins to ossify are between the calcaneus and talus (around 8 to 12 years of age) and between the calcaneaus and navicular bones (around 12 to 16 years).[3] It is thought that microfractures in a coalition cause the pain. Presenting pain may be insidious in onset or initiated with an ankle sprain.

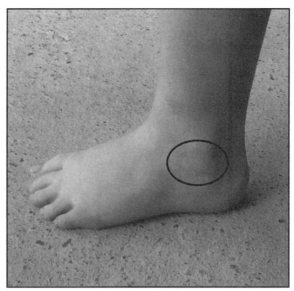

Figure 19-2. Area where isolated tenderness or swelling occurs that does not require a radiograph.

The pain is often aggravated by sports activity or walking on uneven ground. Clinical examination may find pain on palpation over the coalition, restriction of subtalar or calcaneonavicular joint motion, or tight peroneal muscles that resist inversion. A major sign is the failure of the calcaneus to invert during a heel raise or, in children with flat feet, the failure of the arch to be restored during a heel raise.[4] Radiographs may show the coalition, however magnetic resonance imaging (MRI) is considered to be the investigation of choice in pediatric patients.

Osteochondral lesions mostly occur in adolescents. The mechanism of injury is similar to that of an ankle sprain but with a compressive element such as landing from a jump. Presenting pain is usually in the anterior ankle region and has often built up from intermittent pain to an unremitting ache. It is not unusual for the child's symptoms to deteriorate after an initial period of improvement with correct rehabilitation. Palpation will elicit pain over the talar dome but not over the ankle ligaments. Ankle joint motion, particularly dorsiflexion, is typically restricted. If an osteochondral injury is suspected, MRI or isotope bone scanning should be conducted.[4]

The presence of a cavus foot type in conjunction with recurrent sprains, trips, or falls should result in a thorough neurologic examination. CMT disease, the most prevalent childhood peripheral neuropathy, may present in children for the first time in this way. The peripheral neuropathy causes selective weakness in the lower leg resulting typically in lateral ankle instability and foot posture changes toward pes cavus. Clinical examination may reveal decreased dorsiflexion range of motion, sensory loss, and weakness in comparison to healthy children. Decreased eversion to inversion and dorsiflexion to plantar flexion strength ratios may also be present.

Overall, there should be no difference in the clinical examination techniques of the pediatric ankle from that of the adult ankle. Different developmental stages increase the suspicion of fractures rather than sprain in children with an acute injury and the presence of other conditions with chronic ankle problems.

Conclusion

The clinical evaluation may be the same for the pediatric and adult ankle; however, the list of probable differential diagnoses can differ. On the basis of the information presented here, an ankle sprain in the pediatric patient may not be "just a sprain."

References

1. Doherty C, Delahunt E, Caulfield B, et al. The incidence and prevalence of ankle sprain injury: a systematic review and meta-analysis of prospective epidemiological studies. *Sports Med.* 2014:44:123-140.
2. Boutis K, Grootendorst P, Willan A, et al. Effect of the low risk ankle rule on the frequency of radiography in children with ankle injuries. *CMAJ.* 2013:185:E731-E738.
3. Kraft D, Zippin J. Pediatric problems and rehabilitation geared to the young athlete. In Porter DA, Schon LC, eds. *Baxter's The Foot and Ankle in Sport.* Philadelphia, PA: Mosby Elsevier; 2008:535-546.
4. Burns J, Redmond AC, Hunt J. *Childhood Disorders of the Foot and Lower Limb.* New York: Nova Science Publishers Inc; 2012.

SECTION III

TREATMENT AND REHABILITATION

SHOULD I IMMOBILIZE AND RESTRICT WEIGHT BEARING FOR AN ACUTE ANKLE SPRAIN AND, IF SO, WITH WHAT AND FOR HOW LONG?

Tricia Hubbard-Turner, PhD, ATC, FACSM

Initial management of lateral ankle sprains (LAS) typically consists of a combination of rest, ice, compression, and elevation (RICE). After this immediate management, functional rehabilitation is included as part of the rehabilitation plan. Unfortunately, the high percentage of reinjury occurrence (up to 70%)[1] and development of chronic ankle instability suggests that current techniques alone may not be adequate. Hubbard and Cordova[2] measured ankle laxity (anterior displacement and inversion/eversion rotation) 3 days after an LAS and again 8 weeks after injury. They reported that ankle laxity did not significantly decrease over 8 weeks after an acute LAS (Table 20-1).[2] The subjects in this study were instructed to follow basic RICE management during the acute phase and then were given basic functional exercises (range of motion, strengthening, balance) to do. The lack of immobilization and restricted weight bearing may be the reason that subjects had significantly more ankle laxity than those in a control group both immediately after the sprain and again 8 weeks after injury.

The study by Hubbard and Cordova[2] demonstrated the need to examine initial ankle sprain treatment and management more effectively. The residual laxity reported in their study may lead to changes in joint biomechanics and

McKeon PO, Wikstrom EA, eds. *Quick Questions in Ankle Sprains: Expert Advice in Sports Medicine* (pp 103-106).
© 2015 SLACK Incorporated.

Table 20-1

Means and Standard Deviations of Laxity 3 Days and 8 Weeks After Injury

	3 Days After Injury		8 Weeks After Injury	
	Involved Ankle	Uninvolved Ankle	Matched Ankle	Uninvolved Ankle
Anterior displacement (mm)	15.27 + 1.5*	9.79 + .84*	14.18 + 1.1*	9.73 + 1.1*
Inversion rotation (degrees)	36.68 + 3.1**	32.55 + 3.4**	34.67 + 3.5**	32.6 + 3.3**

* Significant difference between the involved ankle and the uninvolved ankle of the injured group ($P = .001$).

** Significant difference between the involved ankle and the uninvolved ankle of the injured group ($P = .047$).

neuromuscular control, all of which may lead to the development of chronic ankle instability. By examining initial management to ensure that ligament healing occurs after injury, long-term disability may be avoided. Beynnon et al[3] were one of the first groups to study long-term (6 months after sprain) outcomes after an ankle sprain secondary to the type of immobilization subjects were given. In this study, subjects received treatment on the basis of the grade (I, II, or III) of ankle sprain they suffered. The authors used the grading scale described by Bergfeld et al.[4] A grade I injury included a partial tear of the lateral ligament complex; a grade II sprain involved decreased motion and some loss of function, a torn anterior talofibular ligament, and an intact calcaneofibular ligament. The subjects would demonstrate positive anterior drawer and negative talar tilt test results. For a grade III sprain, there was almost total loss of function and a complete tear of the lateral ligament complex, as evidenced by positive anterior drawer and talar tilt test results. In addition to the 10-day immobilization, all sprains received a standardized functional rehabilitation protocol. The authors compared an elastic wrap (current standard of care), Air-Stirrup ankle brace, Air-Stirrup ankle brace with an elastic wrap, and fiberglass walking cast. They reported that treatment of grade I and grade II ankle sprains with the Air-Stirrup brace combined with elastic wrap allowed patients to return to their preinjury function quicker than treatment with the other immobilizers.[3] For grade III sprains, there were no differences between the Air-Stirrup brace combined with elastic wrap and the fiberglass walking cast. On the basis of these results, subjects with ankle sprains (even minor ones) should be treated with more stringent immobilization to help with return to activity than with the current standard of care: an elastic wrap. The study did not measure ankle

Table 20-2	
Recommended Immobilization Based on Grade of Ankle Sprain	
Grade I sprain	Air-Stirrup ankle brace with an elastic wrap
Grade II sprain	Air-Stirrup ankle brace with an elastic wrap
Grade III sprain	Below-the-knee cast

laxity, so it is not known if there were differences in the stability of the ankle based on the type of immobilization.

More recently, a multicenter prospective randomized control trial was conducted to examine 3 different supports (Aircast brace, Bledsoe boot, and a 10-day below-knee cast) compared with a double-layer tubular compression bandage (current standard of care) in promoting recovery during the first 9 months after severe LAS.[5] A severe ankle sprain was classified by the patient being unable to bear weight for at least 3 days after the injury. Patients who received a below-knee cast had a more rapid recovery than those who were given the tubular compression bandage. There were clinically important benefits in quality of ankle function 3 months after injury.[5] Bledsoe boots were reported to be the least effective treatment throughout the recovery period. The authors reported that a short period of immobilization in a below-knee cast or Aircast ankle brace may result in faster recovery than the current standard of care. Additionally, the authors recommended the below-knee cast because it showed the widest range of benefit. Unfortunately, this study relied primarily on subjective function, and ankle laxity and subsequent ankle injuries were not measured. However, the evidence from this study does support the need for sturdier immobilization. The subjects in the study by Lamb et al[5] were considered to have severe ankle sprains, which may be why they reported the below-knee cast as most favorable. In less severe sprains (grades I and II), less stringent immobilization like an Air-Stirrup brace combined with elastic wrap may best restore function.

On the basis of the current research evidence, a more sturdy form of immobilization, relative to an elastic wrap alone, is needed to help patients return to function (Table 20-2). The length of time they are immobilized should be based on the healing response of tissues. By having a sturdier form of immobilization, the stress placed on newly laid down tissue can be controlled to ensure that it is not disrupted. This may facilitate greater tissue healing, restoring joint stability, and the patient's ability to return to normal function. Future research should examine ankle laxity with different types of immobilization to confirm if that is the mechanism behind the better subjective function and return to activity reported in the studies. Currently, there have been no randomized trials examining weight-bearing status and its effect on tissue healing and restoration of function. Further research is necessary to examine if there is a non-weight-bearing time that is most beneficial for facilitating tissue healing with immobilization, which will allow clinicians to make evidence-based decisions to help reduce the development of chronic ankle instability.

References

1. Yeung MS, Chan KM, So CH, Yuan WY. An epidemiological survey on ankle sprain. *Br J Sports Med*. 1994;28:112-116.
2. Hubbard TJ, Cordova ML. Mechanical instability after an acute lateral ankle sprain. *Arch Phys Med Rehabil*. 2009a;90:1142-1146.
3. Beynnon BD, Renstrom PA, Haugh L, Uh BS, Barker H. A prospective, randomized clinical investigation of the treatment of first-time ankle sprains. *Am J Sports Med*. 2006;34:1401-1412.
4. Bergfeld J, Cox J, Drez D, et al. Symposium: management of acute ankle sprains. *Contemp Orthop*. 1986;13:83-116.
5. Lamb SE, Marsh JL, Nakash R, Cooke MW. Mechanical supports for acute, severe ankle sprain: a pragmatic, multicentre, randomised controlled trial. *Lancet*. 2009;373:575-581.

WHAT IS THE MOST IMPORTANT IMMEDIATE TREATMENT FOLLOWING AN ANKLE SPRAIN?

Michael G. Dolan, MA, ATC, CSCS

Immediate Care

The immediate care of ankle sprains remains centered on the clinical concepts of protection, rest, ice, compression, and elevation (PRICE). PRICE is almost universally accepted as the clinical gold standard for immediate care of ankle sprains and other soft-tissue injuries. The primary goals of PRICE are to reduce pain, swelling, and secondary tissue damage and to hasten recovery. While there are very few high-quality clinical trials supporting individual components of PRICE or the cumulative effect of all components of the treatment paradigm,[1] there is clear clinical consensus on the use of PRICE.

Immediately following an ankle sprain, the application of ice, compression, and elevation (ICE) should be simultaneously applied as soon as possible after the injury (Table 21-1). Cryotherapy can be applied in a variety of modes, but a plastic bag filled with crushed ice is simple and inexpensive. The bag should be placed directly on the skin over the injury site and surrounding area for 20 to 30 minutes. This time interval was challenged by Bleakley et al,[2] who compared a 20-minute treatment with two 10-minute treatments separated by a 10-minute rest period; they found that the intermittent treatment produced less pain 1 week following injury but reported no differences in swelling and subjective function. Currently,

McKeon PO, Wikstrom EA, eds. *Quick Questions in Ankle Sprains: Expert Advice in Sports Medicine* (pp 107-111). © 2015 SLACK Incorporated.

Table 21-1
Immediate Care of Ankle Sprains

Time Following Injury	Interventions	Comments
0 to 60 minutes	Two 20- to 30-minute bouts of ice, compression, and elevation interspersed by a clinical reevaluation	If clinical evaluation indicates fracture via Ottawa rules, obtain radiograph
60 minutes to 24 hours	Application of compression and stirrup brace to restrict inversion/eversion; instruct athlete to apply ice, compression, and elevation for pain as needed; clinical guidelines and practicality suggest this occurs every 1 to 2 hours	Apply as needed for pain management or significant movement event such as walking to dormitory, returning from class, etc
60 minutes to 24 hours	Joint mobilizations for pain and limiting restrictions in joint motion	Appropriate training in joint mobilization techniques is required
After injury	NSAIDS	At discretion of physician

the optimal mode, duration, and frequency of reapplication have not been established, so most treatment parameters are based on expert opinion and clinical consensus.[1] The primary benefit of cryotherapy is analgesia, and it should be reapplied as needed. Current practice suggests reapplication every 1 to 2 hours or when pain increases and after a significant movement event, such as returning home after the injury. Caution should be used when applying chemical cold packs, and they should not be applied directly to the skin because temperatures are below freezing and direct exposure to the skin can cause tissue damage. Therefore, a wet paper towel or other barrier should be placed between the skin and gel pack if other forms of cryotherapy are not available.

During the initial ICE application, the ice pack should be held in place with an elastic bandage (Figure 21-1). The bandage not only secures the ice bag against the skin but also produces compression on the injury site. Compression increases hydrostatic pressure at the injury site and counteracts the increased osmotic pressure resulting from the injury, which is the primary cause of edema formation following ankle sprains. Although compression is almost universally accepted, the optimal mode and duration of use following ankle sprains have not been established.

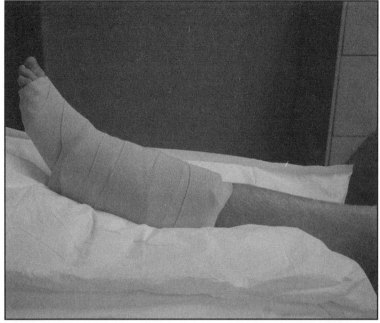

Figure 21-1. Application of ice, compression, and elevation following an acute ankle sprain.

The final component of the initial ICE intervention is elevation. The injured limb should be elevated as high as possible within the physical limitations of the patient; a minimum of 45 degrees is suggested. Elevation decreases hydrostatic pressure at the injury site and encourages lymphatic drainage.

Follow-Up Care

Following the initial ICE treatment, the limb should be compressed with elastic wrap, starting at the toes and extending up to the midcalf. An alternative is the use of a commercial compression sleeve. In addition, some clinicians use focal compression, which is the application of a foam or felt horseshoe pad that is placed over the sites with the most swelling. In theory, the additional material inhibits edema formation by adding additional pressure over the sinus tarsi, the most common location of swelling following lateral ankle sprains. Research comparing different modes of compression has not established a true gold standard, so clinical judgment is required.

After compression is applied, the ankle should be protected with a stirrup-type brace. The brace applies additional compression and allows the patient to bear weight as tolerated. The brace allows ankle dorsiflexion and plantar flexion but restricts inversion and eversion. The combination of compression, bracing, and

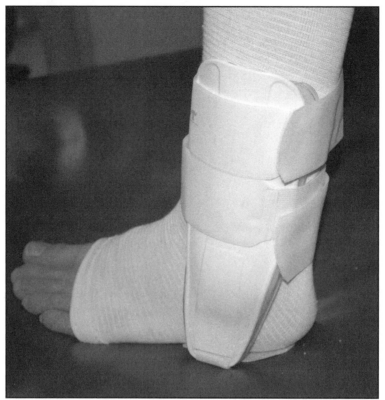

Figure 21-2. Use of a compression sleeve and brace during the acute phase of injury.

gradual weight bearing and exercise is termed *functional rehabilitation* and is the current gold standard for rehabilitation of grade I and II lateral ankle sprains.[3] If the patient is unable to walk without pain and/or functional impairment, he or she should be fitted for crutches, and further forms of protection/immobilization may be necessary (Figure 21-2).

Other Interventions

Some clinicians supplement PRICE with other interventions to manage acute ankle sprains. Nonsteroidal anti-inflammatory drugs (NSAIDs) during the acute and subacute phases of injury decrease pain and improve short-term function following acute ankle sprains. However, this practice is not without controversy, and the decision to use NSAIDS should be made in consultation with the attending physician. Although the short-term pain relief is clear, some are concerned that it may lead to incomplete healing and have suggested that administration of NSAIDs may result in reduced strength of healed tendons and ligaments and may, therefore, make those structures more liable to future injuries.[4]

Joint mobilizations have been an integral part of ankle rehabilitation for years but are seldom considered an acute intervention. Green et al[5] reported that the addition of anteroposterior joint mobilization to a standard RICE protocol improved dorsiflexion range of motion and gait compared to a group that received RICE alone. In addition, gentle joint mobilizations are frequently used to modulate pain during the acute phase of injury.

The most important treatment following an acute ankle sprain is the application of PRICE. Immediately following injury, the management of pain and the other components of the inflammatory process is critical. Immediate care should be considered the first step in a comprehensive rehabilitation program and should be applied as quickly after injury as possible (see Table 21-1).

References

1. van der Bekerom MP, Struijs PA, Blankevoort L, et al. What is the evidence for rest, ice, compression, and elevation therapy in the treatment of ankle sprains in adults? *J Athl Train.* 2012;47:435-443.
2. Bleakley CM, McDonough SM, MacAuley DC. Cryotherapy for acute ankle sprains: a randomised controlled study of two different icing protocols. *Br J Sports Med.* 2006;40:700-705.
3. Beynnon BD, Renstrom PA, Haugh L, Uh BS, Barker H. A prospective, randomized clinical investigation of the treatment of first-time ankle sprains. *Am J Sports Med.* 2006;34:1401-1412.
4. Mishra DK, Fridén J, Schmitz MC, Lieber RL. Anti-inflammatory medication after muscle injury: a treatment resulting in short-term improvement but subsequent loss of muscle function. *J Bone Joint Surg Am.* 1995;77:1510-1519.
5. Green T, Refshauge K, Crosbie J, Adams R. A randomized controlled trial of a passive accessory joint mobilization on acute ankle inversion sprains. *Phys Ther.* 2001;81:984-994.

WHAT ARE THE MOST IMPORTANT COMPONENTS TO INCLUDE IN A REHABILITATION PROGRAM FOLLOWING AN ANKLE SPRAIN?

Scott E. Ross, PhD, LAT, ATC, FNATA
and Brent L. Arnold, PhD, ATC, FNATA

Ankle sprains are common injuries occurring with physical activity. As result, a great need exists to use evidence-based medicine to rehabilitate sprains to prevent reinjury episodes. Therapeutic exercise is one component of a treatment program that should be implemented to manage these sprains.[1] More specifically, experts recently recommended in a position statement for the treatment of ankle sprains that clinicians need to treat sprains with therapeutic exercises that focus on range of motion, strength, and sensorimotor function.[1] Interestingly, however, clinical research trials on acute ankle sprains are not abundant in the literature, and the few results that do exist demonstrate only some degree of evidence for reducing reinjury following the rehabilitation of acute ankle sprains with therapeutic exercises.[2,3] Evidence in the literature also establishes that clinical impairments in edema, strength, and balance can be corrected with interventions[1]; however, edema, strength, and balance can also return to normal without supervised or formalized rehabilitation.[2,3] Consequently, our focus for this chapter is to recommend the inclusion of specific therapeutic exercises associated with ankle sprain reinjury reduction following a rehabilitation program for acute ankle sprain.[2-5] We first

McKeon PO, Wikstrom EA, eds. *Quick Questions in
Ankle Sprains: Expert Advice in Sports Medicine* (pp 113-117).
© 2015 SLACK Incorporated.

outline the appropriate exercises to administer and provide supporting evidence for their effectiveness in reducing reinjuries, and then we outline frequency and volume parameters for rehabilitation programs.

Therapeutic Exercises

RANGE OF MOTION AND STRENGTH

We encourage clinicians to include range-of-motion and strengthening exercises in rehabilitation programs to reduce ankle sprain reinjury incidences. Common exercises on which to focus in rehabilitation are active ankle/foot circumduction,[3,5] isolated active plantar flexion/dorsiflexion,[5] diagonal movement patterns of the ankle/foot,[5] and triceps surae static stretch.[5] Open kinetic chain isometric strengthening exercises for eversion, inversion, dorsiflexion, and plantar flexion should be included in the first few weeks following injury.[5] Furthermore, strengthening can be performed in a closed kinetic chain on a flat surface by performing toe raises and heel raises.[3] To progress the rehabilitation, heel raises off of an elevated platform can be initiated by first allowing patients to hold onto a structure and then progress to performing this exercise without stability assistance.[4] Last, patients can perform isometric strengthening by standing on both legs on the outside of the feet (supination) and then switch to standing on the inside of the feet (pronation).[3] This type of closed kinetic chain exercise can be performed first with eyes opened and then progress to doing it with eyes closed.[3]

SENSORIMOTOR TRAINING

Sensorimotor training in the form of double-leg and single-leg balance exercises on level surfaces and wobble boards are most commonly used in rehabilitation to prevent ankle sprain reinjury.[2-4] In a very basic form, clinicians can have patients perform a double-leg stance on a wobble board with anterior/posterior rocks, medial/lateral rocks, and circumduction.[2] In both types of rocking, patients should not allow the edges of the wobble board to touch the ground.[2] Patients can begin these wobble board exercises with the eyes opened and progress to doing them with the eyes closed and then progress from a relatively straight-leg stance to a stance with more knee flexion.[2] Wobble board exercises also can be advanced to single-leg stances with the eyes opened and eyes closed.[3] Standing on a single leg on a wobble board and playing ball toss are also useful in rehabilitation protocols.[3]

More complex exercises on wobble boards can be added to the rehabilitation but generally require a progression by beginning the exercises on level surfaces, performing exercises with and without vision, and then using wobble boards.[4] Four exercises have been recommended with this type of progression.[4] The first exercise position is standing on a single leg, and then flexion of the stance leg should commence while swinging the non-weight-bearing leg into extension with simultaneous movement of the ipsilateral arm to the non-weight-bearing leg into flexion (return to starting position and repeat).[4] Next a simple single-leg stance can be performed with the non-weight-bearing hip extended, knee flexed, and foot held slightly off of the floor.[4] This position should be held for 1 minute and then repeated.[4] A progression off of this exercise is to perform a single-leg stance and then begin swinging the non-weight-bearing leg into hip flexion with the knee flexed and simultaneously swinging the contralateral arm to the non-weight-bearing leg into flexion (return to starting position and repeat).[4] Finally, patients can perform a single-leg stance and begin swinging the non-weight-bearing leg into adduction with the toes pointed and then swinging it back into abduction with the toes pointed (return to starting position and repeat).[4] Patients may need to begin this exercise while touching a structure for added stability.[4]

FUNCTIONAL MOVEMENT

A few functional movement exercises also have been recommended for rehabilitation programs. Figure 8 running and hopping on one foot are 2 exercises that clinicians can add to their protocols.[3] Walking with the heels off of the ground (on tiptoes) with the foot in various positions is recommended.[4] Patients can walk 4 m with the foot in neutral (toes forward), turn around and walk back 4 m with the foot rotated outward, and then turn around one last time and walk 4 m with the foot rotated inward.[4] This exercise can be repeated with the same foot positions and distance traveled, except patients can perform double-legged jumps instead of walking.[4]

Diagnostic Parameters

We computed the risk of sustaining an ankle sprain following interventions (statistically known as relative risk) and the effectiveness of interventions for preventing sprains (statistically known as number need to treat) from 3 investigations that examined the treatment effects of acute ankle rehabilitation on reducing ankle sprain reinjury (Table 22-1). These diagnostic statistics were computed to categorize the strength of each treatment effect. (Values closer to 0% are considered strong.) The risks of sustaining an ankle sprain following therapeutic interventions in the 3 studies reviewed were 18%,[3] 46%,[2] and 65%[4]; thus, the risk of sustaining an ankle sprain reinjury following exposure to rehabilitation are low[3] to moderate.[2,4] To make these diagnostic statistics more clinically meaningful, we determined the effectiveness of the interventions to determine how many individuals must be

Table 22-1

Frequency and Effectiveness of Training

Study	Relative Risk Ratio (95% CI) (Risk of Sustaining a Sprain)	Number Needed to Treat (Effectiveness of Treatment)	Minutes/ Session	Sessions/ Week	Weeks in Training	Volume
Wester et al[2]	0.46 (0.21 to 1.01)[†]	3[†]	15	7	12	21
Holme et al[3]	0.18 (0.04 to 0.78)[‡]	5[‡]	60	2	6	12
Hupperets et al[4]	0.65 (0.50 to 0.87)	9	30	3	8	12
Bleakley et al[5]	*	*	30	Not reported	4	2

CI = confidence interval.

*We did not compute relative risk ratio or number needed to treat for Bleakley et al[5] because the control group had the same treatment as the experimental group, but it was delayed by 1 week.

†Wester et al findings are not statistically significant because the relative risk value of the 95% CI crosses 1. However, we consider these results clinically meaningful because the statistics are influenced by the low sample size.

‡We did not control for exposure. Hupperets et al[4] did control for exposure, but we computed the relative risk ratio from their study without controlling for exposure to match the other 2 studies (which did not control for exposure).

exposed to rehabilitation to prevent one ankle sprain reinjury. Depending on the type of rehabilitation, our calculations reveal that 3,[2] 5,[3] or 9[4] ankle sprains need to be rehabilitated to prevent one ankle sprain reinjury (see Table 22-1). Thus, lower values (eg, 3) indicate that the treatment is more effective than those with higher values (eg, 9).

It is worth noting that supervised rehabilitation is an important factor to consider in treating ankle sprains, because it lowers the risk of ankle sprains to 18%.[3] Rehabilitation programs that have patients perform exercises outside of a treatment facility have only moderate reduction in ankle sprains.[2,4] Beginning exercises during the first stage or early second stage of healing will result in similar reductions in ankle sprain reinjury.[5] However, waiting to commence rehabilitation in the later second stages or early third stages of healing may not be as effective in preventing sprains[4] than beginning in the early stages.[2,3]

Frequency and Volume of Treatment

We also want to provide guidance for the frequency and volume of training for rehabilitation based on the evidence that was reviewed in the literature. We provide data on the frequency and volume of training from the investigations that we have reviewed in this chapter (see Table 22-1). On the basis of these data, our recommendation is for clinicians to design rehabilitation programs that require patients to perform rehabilitation in 34-minute training sessions, 4 times per week, for a minimum of 8 weeks. This recommendation provides a volume of 18 hours.

Conclusion

Evidence is available to demonstrate that therapeutic exercise has relevance in rehabilitation programs for reducing ankle sprain reinjury episodes. We first recommend that rehabilitation take place under the supervision of a sports medicine clinician. Second, acute ankle sprain exercises for rehabilitation should include range of motion, strengthening, sensorimotor training, and functional movement. Sensorimotor training can emphasize balance training with and without wobble boards. Finally, we recommend that patients perform rehabilitation in 34-minute training sessions, 4 times per week, for a minimum of 8 weeks to maximize the effectiveness of the intervention in reducing ankle sprains.

References

1. Kaminski TW, Hertel J, Amendola N, et al. National Athletic Trainers' Association position statement: conservative management and prevention of ankle sprains in athletes. *J Athl Train*. 2013;48:528-545.
2. Wester JU, Jespersen SM, Nielsen KD, Neumann L. Wobble board training after partial sprains of the lateral ligaments of the ankle: a prospective randomized study. *J Orthop Sport Phys Ther*. 1996;23:332-336.
3. Holme E, Magnusson SP, Becher K, et al. The effect of supervised rehabilitation on strength, postural sway, position sense and re-injury risk after acute ligament sprain. *Scand J Med Sci Sports*. 1999;9:104.
4. Hupperets MD, Verhagen EA, van Mechelen W. Effect of unsupervised home based proprioceptive training on recurrences of ankle sprain: randomised controlled trial. *Br Med J*. 2009;339:b2684.
5. Bleakley CM, O'Connor SR, Tully MA, et al. Effect of accelerated rehabilitation on function after ankle sprain: randomised controlled trial. *Br Med J*. 2010;340:c1964.

WHAT TREATMENTS ARE MOST EFFECTIVE FOR INCREASING DORSIFLEXION DURING THE REHABILITATION PROCESS, AND HOW LONG SHOULD I EXPECT DORSIFLEXION DEFICITS TO BE PRESENT IN MY PATIENT?

Patrick O. McKeon, PhD, ATC, CSCS
and Erik A. Wikstrom, PhD, ATC, FACSM

It is well known that lateral ankle sprains are one of the most common injuries associated with physical activity. The most common mechanism for these injuries is a combination of plantar flexion and inversion/supination resulting in damage to the anterior talofibular and calcaneofibular ligaments. The damage to these ligaments results in increased anterior translation of the talus and increased subtalar motion in the frontal plane. While these 2 issues are commonly reported, a major resulting issue that has received increased attention recently is a deficit in dorsiflexion. Dorsiflexion deficits in those with ankle instability appear to be the result of the arthrokinematic alterations associated with the damage to the corresponding ankle ligaments mentioned earlier. This is referred to as a talar positional fault.[1] Because of acute damage, the anterior talofibular ligament no longer provides adequate restriction of anterior talar glide, and thus, the talus has an

McKeon PO, Wikstrom EA, eds. *Quick Questions in Ankle Sprains: Expert Advice in Sports Medicine* (pp 119-122).
© 2015 SLACK Incorporated.

increased tendency to develop a slightly anterior position in relation to the mortise. This positional fault then translates to a decrease in posterior talar glide, which is coupled with a decrease in dorsiflexion. Dorsiflexion plays a vital role in the ability to absorb force during weight-bearing activities and has a direct influence on knee and hip range of motion. A dorsiflexion deficit because of ankle instability can certainly contribute to an increased likelihood of recurring ankle sprain because of the altered position of the talus and the impaired ability to absorb force. Addressing the talar arthrokinematic restriction to prevent the development of a dorsiflexion deficit should be a top priority in ankle sprain rehabilitation. Several techniques for enhancing dorsiflexion after ankle sprain have been described in the literature, including joint mobilization, traction with high-velocity low-amplitude manipulation, and stretching. The purpose of this chapter is to discuss the most effective rehabilitation strategies for enhancing dorsiflexion via arthrokinematic impairments or calf muscle tightness.

To address the arthrokinematic restrictions related to dorsiflexion in those with chronic ankle instability (CAI), several treatment techniques have been shown to be effective. Ankle joint mobilizations using a Maitland technique in which a therapist employs large-amplitude anterior-to-posterior talar oscillations to move the patient's talus through the range of arthrokinematic motion to the posterior joint restriction have been shown to increase dorsiflexion in as few as one treatment. This type of mobilization is performed while the patient is sitting on a treatment table and the therapist moves the talus on the tibia. In a recent study, Hoch et al[2] found that two 2-minute sets of these mobilizations substantially increased dorsiflexion as measured through the weight-bearing lunge test in those with CAI. When this technique was employed over the course of 2 weeks (3 treatments per week) in this patient population, the dorsiflexion increase was 3-fold that of the control group and was maintained at least for 2 weeks after treatment. It is apparent that Maitland ankle joint mobilizations can enhance dorsiflexion in those with CAI. However, no investigation to date has quantified the effectiveness of calf muscle stretching on dorsiflexion deficits in those with the CAI.

Although acute ankle sprains and CAI are injury issues in the same joint, treatment strategies for enhancing dorsiflexion are slightly different. Multiple treatments of small-amplitude oscillations have been shown to enhance dorsiflexion over the course of 2 weeks in patients with acute sprains. However, a single treatment of joint mobilizations was not shown to improve dorsiflexion beyond that of rest, ice, compression, and elevation in those patients who had suffered an acute ankle sprain,[3] unlike the results observed in those with CAI. This is an important consideration, as one treatment may not be enough for acute ankle sprains. Rather, multiple treatments of joint mobilizations (approximately 6 treatment sessions over the course of 2 weeks) seem to be most appropriate. Additionally, techniques such as passive calf stretching and mobilization with movement (MWM) have demonstrated improvements in dorsiflexion in those with acute ankle sprains and CAI.[4] Last, for acute ankle sprains with calf muscle tightness, calf stretching appears to be a good avenue for increasing dorsiflexion range of motion. Having patients perform 3 stretches over the course of the day held anywhere from 30 seconds to 2 minutes increases dorsiflexion beyond rest, ice, compression, and elevation over the course of 2 to 6 weeks.[3] It may be that spasm within the calf muscles due to ankle sprain restricts dorsiflexion. Calf stretching with static holds appears to reduce this type of dorsiflexion restriction. When considering enhancing dorsiflexion as a treatment for acute ankle sprains, joint mobilization (either small-amplitude oscillations or MWM) in combination with a calf-stretching program over the course of at least 2 weeks may be the most beneficial strategy, especially when the underlying cause is difficult to identify.

For both CAI and acute ankle sprains, when attempting to restore normal dorsiflexion at the ankle, it is important to ensure that the patient's talus can glide on the tibia. Joint traction is very beneficial for this and, in combination with HVLA manipulation or passive mobilization, should be used to distract the talus from the tibia. See Question 30 for a full description of these techniques. Traction in combination with HVLA has been shown to be beneficial for increasing dorsiflexion, but not to the same degree as joint mobilization.[5] The combination of traction and joint mobilization was used in the Hoch et al study mentioned before, which may be one of the reasons for the dramatic increase in dorsiflexion in those with CAI.

There is good evidence to suggest that dorsiflexion deficits are present in those with acute ankle sprains and CAI due to either calf muscle tightness or posterior talar glide deficits. Unfortunately, it remains unclear how long these deficits last. However, patients with CAI seem to demonstrate these deficits fairly consistently, and these individuals are often observed years after their initial injury. Further, these deficits appear to be connected to self-reported functional limitations, which may be a very important issue for which to screen in patients. If a patient reports that he or she feels unstable or limited in activities such as running, cutting, landing, or jumping, take the time to evaluate whether a dorsiflexion restriction, regardless of the cause, is present. Several issues seem to be influential in the development of dorsiflexion deficits, including pain, swelling, perceived stiffness, and a period of immobilization. It is important to include an assessment of dorsiflexion as an outcome measure in the treatment of acute sprains and ankle instability and to keep track of how well a person responds to treatments. For example, if calf stretching is used and no improvements in dorsiflexion are found after 1 week, suspect that the restriction may be coming from a posterior talar glide restriction. Joint mobilizations (either Maitland or MWM) may be the optimal treatment strategy for this type of condition. More than likely, a combination of stretching and joint mobilization is the most appropriate choice for both acute ankle sprains and CAI. From the literature, the sensitive methods of screening for dorsiflexion deficits and/or posterior talar glide restrictions include the weight-bearing lunge test, open-chain active dorsiflexion, and the posterior talar glide test. Keeping the development of dorsiflexion deficits via calf muscle tightness or posterior talar glide restrictions on the clinical radar screen is critically important for the treatment of acute sprains and ankle instability and should be evaluated regularly as a rehabilitation outcome.

References

1. Wikstrom EA, Hubbard TJ. Talar positional fault in persons with chronic ankle instability. *Arch Phys Med Rehabil.* 2010;91:1267-1271.
2. Hoch MC, Andreatta RD, Mullineaux DR, et al. Two-week joint mobilization intervention improves self-reported function, range of motion, and dynamic balance in those with chronic ankle instability. *J Orthop Res.* 2012;30:1798-1804.
3. Terada M, Pietrosimone BG, Gribble PA. Therapeutic interventions for increasing ankle dorsiflexion after ankle sprain: a systematic review. *J Athl Train.* 2013;48:696-709.
4. Loudon JK, Reiman MP, Sylvain J. The efficacy of manual joint mobilisation/manipulation in treatment of lateral ankle sprains: a systematic review. *Br J Sports Med.* 2014;48:365-370.
5. Wikstrom EA, McKeon PO. Manipulative therapy effectiveness following acute lateral ankle sprains: a systematic review. *Athl Train Sports Health Care.* 2011;3:271-279.

WHAT IS CUBOID SYNDROME FOLLOWING TRAUMATIC LATERAL ANKLE SPRAIN, AND HOW SHOULD IT BE TREATED?

Helene Simpson, MSc Physiotherapy

Incidence

Cuboid syndrome is defined as a minor disruption of the structural congruity of the calcaneocuboid (CC) joint complex. It is an often-misdiagnosed complication of a plantar flexion/inversion lateral sprain of the ankle. Cuboid syndrome is uncommon; it is reported in 6.7% of patients with sprains of the lateral ligament complex of the ankle.[1]

Presentation

After the typical symptoms of a lateral ankle sprain (pain localized to the anterior talofibular ligament and calcaneofibular ligament) should have subsided,[2] athletes may complain of a sharp and persistent pain located in the CC-joint area. Pain may also radiate along the lateral border of the foot between the cuboid and the fourth or fifth metatarsals[1,2]; it is often pronounced and aggravated during the push-off

McKeon PO, Wikstrom EA, eds. *Quick Questions in Ankle Sprains: Expert Advice in Sports Medicine* (pp 123-129).
© 2015 SLACK Incorporated.

phase of walking and running. Walking and running over uneven terrain, in which midfoot pronation and supination are accentuated, can also be very painful.[1]

Key clinical features of cuboid syndrome include tenderness to palpation of the peroneus longus tendon along the cuboid groove and the cuboid (both plantar and dorsal aspects)[3], a dropped lateral longitudinal arch, and, most significantly, a slight sulcus on the dorsal aspect of the dorsum of the cuboid and a bony protrusion of the cuboid that can be observed and palpated.[1-3]

Proposed Pathomechanism of Cuboid Syndrome Following a Lateral Ankle Sprain

During a lateral ankle sprain, a subtle subluxation of the cuboid occurs. The mechanism is described as follows:

The intrinsic stability of, and load transfer at, the CC joint during closed-chain activity is facilitated by the action of the peroneus longus tendon. The tendon forms a sling around the lateral and plantar aspects of the cuboid. During mid-stance through to late push off, the cuboid acts as a fulcrum/pulley for the tendon. During an inversion injury, the peroneus longus reflexively contracts to pronate the foot into a more neutral position on the ground.[2] In rare cases, the resultant force subluxes the cuboid as it spins medially around its own axis (along the frontal plane) into the plantar/inferior direction.[2] The structural congruity of the CC complex is thus disrupted, as the cuboid essentially becomes locked out of its functional alignment.[3] A simultaneous disruption/tearing of the interosseous ligaments may occur.[1]

Further Clinical Signs

From the minor loss of congruity of the joint, active and passive longitudinal pronation and supination of the midfoot are limited because of pain in the CC joint. Passive plantar and dorsal glides of the cuboid elicit pain in the CC joint and can reproduce the patient's pain. Swelling may be noted over the CC joint.[1-3]

Differential Diagnosis of Cuboid Syndrome

To date, no definitive, reliable, or valid clinical tests for identifying plantar sub-luxation of the cuboid following a lateral sprain of the ankle have been described.[3] Therefore, the diagnosis is based on key clinical features from the history and signs and symptoms of the injury. To assist diagnosis, see Table 24-1.

Table 24-1
Differential Diagnosis of Cuboid Syndrome Following Lateral Ankle Sprain
Subjective Findings
• Mechanism of injury (plantar flexion and inversion)
• Pain located to cuboid and lateral midfoot
Objective Findings
• Painful palpation of the cuboid
• Antalgic gait (pain during push-off phase)
• Resisted muscle tests—resisted inversion/eversion (pain)
• Passive physiological movements of the midtarsal joint complex—painful symptom reproduction with midtarsal supination and/or midtarsal adduction tests
• Passive accessory movements—painful dorsal glides of the cuboid

The most pertinent signs and symptoms are persistent localized pain and a painful plantar protrusion of the cuboid.[1]

Plain radiographs (according to the Ottawa ankle rules) can rule out fractures.[2] However, radiography, computerized tomography (CT), and magnetic resonance imaging (MRI) have not been found to improve the diagnosis of cuboid syndrome.[3] Diagnostic ultrasound may be useful (before and after treatment), but the evidence is limited to a few reported case studies.[4]

Key diagnoses to rule out before cuboid syndrome can be considered are as follows:

- Fractures of the base of the fifth metatarsal
- Fractures of the cuboid (extremely rare)
- Peroneus longus subluxation and/or tendinopathy
- Nerve root radiculopathy[1-4]

Treatment Options

Cuboid syndrome responds well to treatment, and most athletes return to full function after treatment. Successful treatment modalities include cuboid manipulations, bracing (including foot orthotics), and/or taping combined with comprehensive rehabilitation.

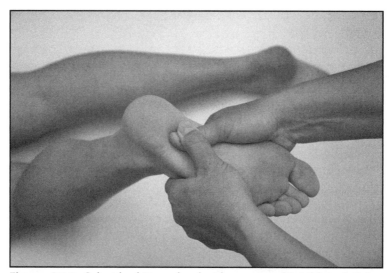

Figure 24-1. Cuboid whip and cuboid squeeze. (1) Athlete is lying prone. Knee is bent to approximately 90 degrees of flexion. (2) Therapist interlocks fingers over the dorsum of the foot to act as a fulcrum, with thumbs positioned over the plantar cuboid (overlapping). (3) Start with ankle in neutral, then exert a dorsally directed, brief, high-velocity, low-amplitude force to the plantar cuboid protrusion while the ankle is swung into full plantar flexion. (4) When performing the squeeze technique; maintain the squeeze while slowing bringing the ankle to full plantar flexion.
Author's suggestion: try to pronate midfoot while swinging into plantar flexion, so the midfoot is relatively "unlocked."

The cuboid whip (Figure 24-1)[1] is the most-cited technique for the treatment of cuboid syndrome/plantar subluxation of the cuboid. In 1992, a modification to the cuboid whip was proposed: the cuboid squeeze. Both of these manipulations are reported to be particularly effective for cuboid syndrome secondary to a lateral ankle sprain.[4] The cuboid squeeze offers the clinician better control and direction of the manipulation and minimizes the amount of force through the injured lateral ligament complex.[1] However, preferred selection of these techniques remains controversial in the absence of published randomized clinical trials.[4]

Another option might be mobilization with movement (MWM),[5] which has been pioneered by Mulligan since the 1970s. This type of mobilization is highly recommended to correct minor positional faults that may cause restrictions of movement and pain, especially after a sprain. Mulligan claimed that with these mobilizations, pain-free, end-of-range function is easily restored and maintained.[5]

The author designed an MWM to relocate the cuboid (Figure 24-2):

- Actively performed limited physiological movement (pronation), with a sustained accessory glide at a right angle to pronation

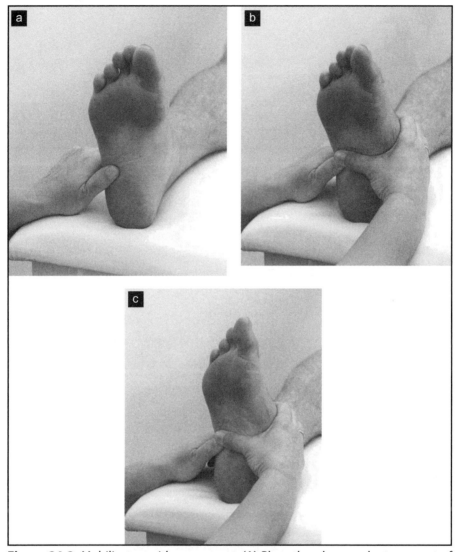

Figure 24-2. Mobilizaton with movement. (A) Place thumb over plantar aspect of cuboid. Apply a dorsal glide to the cuboid and hold. (B) To maintain dorsiflexion, the other hand stabilizes the cuneiform and the medial aspect of the midfoot. (C) While the patient pronates the midfoot, sustain the glide to the end of range (pronation) and back into supination. Pain relief should be immediate. Repeat 6 to 10 times and then reassess for pain.

- Pronation is performed into resistance, but without pain
- To achieve full range of movement, 10 repeats are required

This approach does not put tension on the injured lateral ligaments and/or deep or superficial peroneal nerves. Successful relocation is a painless, audible click of the cuboid. Pain will be immediately reduced, and the limited range of movement

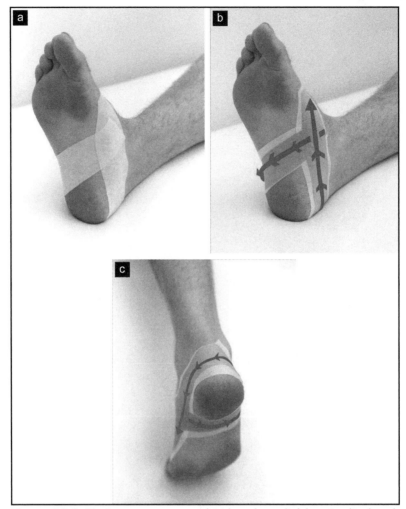

Figure 24-3. Taping to support cuboid and medial longitudinal arch of the ankle-foot complex. (A) Starting at the base of the first metatarsophalangeal joint, apply a strip of cover tape and continue along the medial aspect of the foot; stay inferior to the medial malleolus and the Achilles tendon. (B) Continue around the calcaneus and then around the cuboid toward the medial arch/navicular. (C) Apply a layer of rigid tape to reinforce the cover tape. Note: stand the patient up to test for immediate relief of pain and comfort. Adjust the tape as necessary.

improved.[1-5] If the condition has been present for more than 1 month, the manipulations or MWM may need to be repeated more than once.[2]

Other treatment approaches described in the literature are taping techniques (Figure 24-3) to support the medial arch (to limit excessive pronation) and a cuboid pad on the plantar aspect of the cuboid to prevent plantar gliding.[1-3]

A pain-free rehabilitation regimen should be started immediately after reduction of the cuboid subluxation.[1] Closed kinetic chain exercises are preferred.[4] To improve bilateral and proximal muscular control, proprioception/postural control exercises performed in the stance phase of gait are recommended.[1,4] Strengthening of the intrinsic foot muscles is of great benefit as well.[4]

Patients are advised not to walk barefoot for 4 to 6 weeks. Supportive shoes are advised. The cuboid position should be monitored weekly during this stage.[4]

Cortisone injections are recommended only when pain and inflammation of the injured ligaments and capsule of the CC joint fail to improve. Surgery should be considered as a last resort only, except in cases where there is a recurring instability.[4]

Conclusion

Recognizing cuboid syndrome as a complication following a lateral ankle sprain is important. Once the clinician is familiar with the typical clinical features, the actual diagnosis is easy. The treatment techniques, inclusive of specific joint mobilizations/manipulations proposed in the literature, are safe and cost-effective. Pain relief following the joint mobilizations is almost immediate, and athletes should be able return to sport without recurrence of the injury.[1-4]

References

1. Patterson SM. Cuboid syndrome: a review of the literature. *J Sports Sci Med.* 2006;5:597-606.
2. Jennings J, Davies GJ. Treatment of cuboid syndrome secondary to lateral ankle sprains: a case series. *J Orthop Sports Phys Ther.* 2005;35:409-415.
3. Durall CJ. Examination and treatment of cuboid syndrome: a literature review. *Sports Health.* 2011;3:514-519.
4. Adams E, Madden C. Cuboid subluxation: a case study and review of the literature. *Curr Sports Med Rep.* 2009;8:300-307.
5. Vincenzino B, Paungmali A, Teys P. Mulligan's mobilization-with-movement, positional faults and pain relief: current concepts from a critical review of the literature. *Man Ther.* 2007;12:98-108.

WHAT CRITERIA SHOULD I USE TO RETURN AN ATHLETE TO SPORT AFTER AN ACUTE LATERAL ANKLE SPRAIN?

Chris M. Bleakley, PhD, BSc and Philip Glasgow, PhD, BSc

Ankle sprains commonly occur in sports, with incidence figures ranging between 6.9 and 13.6 injuries per 1000 exposures.[1] Although ankle sprains are often regarded as simple injuries, a large proportion of people suffer chronic pain and instability. Athletes seem to be particularly prone to recurrent problems, with around 33% suffering reinjury when they return to sport.[2]

It is often difficult to determine when an athlete is ready to return to competition after an ankle sprain. Traditionally, return-to-play decisions were informed largely by the absence of pain or the time since injury. This approach often risked a premature return to sport, particularly in circumstances with significant coaching pressure or an overzealous athlete. The current gold standard is to outline sports-specific criteria and functional goals that must be achieved prior to returning to sport. This is a graded, goal-orientated approach in which athletes earn the right to compete by achieving the requisite level of functional performance.[3] We discuss here key criteria that can be used to inform return-to-sport decisions following an ankle sprain.

McKeon PO, Wikstrom EA, eds. *Quick Questions in Ankle Sprains: Expert Advice in Sports Medicine* (pp 131-134).
© 2015 SLACK Incorporated.

Absence of Signs and Symptoms

The presence of pain or giving way should automatically contraindicate a return to sport. These symptoms may be indicative of incomplete anatomical and/or functional healing; practitioners should also consider the possibility that concomitant injuries are present (eg, osteochondral damage, syndesmotic involvement), particularly if significant time has elapsed since the injury (more than 4 to 6 weeks).

The ideal is for swelling to have completely resolved prior to returning to sport. However, as the vasculature at the foot and ankle are subjected to high intravenous pressures, small pockets of persistent swelling can often accumulate around the lateral ankle gutter. This is distinguishable from acute inflammation and is usually unimportant. A reduction in swelling with exercise provides further reassurance of its trivial nature. Vigilance is advised if the athlete presents with posterior or circumferential swelling or if swelling increases significantly after exercise.

The anterior drawer and talar tilt tests are commonly used to assess lateral ankle joint stability. The absence of pain during these tests is an important prerequisite for returning to sport. It is more difficult to provide an optimal threshold for stability. We must consider the possibility that athletes who are managed conservatively will rarely return to their preinjury levels of mechanical stability. Clinical tests of stability are usually interpreted dichotomously (pass/fail); however, a short ordinal scale (stability, mild instability, moderate instability, gross instability) may be more informative for return-to-play decisions. Stability or mild instability is preferable. Returning to play with moderate or gross instability is questionable and requires significant justification.

Adequate Flexibility and Strength

Ankle sprains can cause an anterior shift of the talus, altering the joint's arthrokinematics and restricting ankle dorsiflexion. Athletes who fail to regain full ankle dorsiflexion after an ankle injury seem to be at an increased risk of injury. Dorsiflexion can be reliably assessed using a weight-bearing lunge test. A simple bilateral squat test provides additional information on dynamic flexibility at the ankle joint. Athletes should be able to squat symmetrically and without pain. Be aware that heel lifting, overpronation, or weight-shifting are commonly used to compensate for dorsiflexion limitations. The single-leg calf raise test is often used to quantify the work capacity of the triceps surae muscle complex. After an ankle sprain, it is useful to modify this test as outlined in Figure 25-1; here the athlete must complete the calf-raise test while ensuring that the ball of his or her foot does

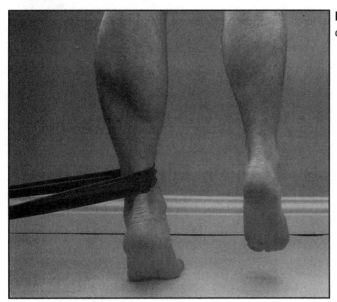

Figure 25-1. Modified single-leg calf-raise test.

not lift from the ground. This incorporates the peroneal muscle group, including the peroneus longus, which has an important role in preventing excessive supination.

Functional Fitness and Sports-Specific Skills

A key criterion is determining whether the athlete has regained the requisite functional and technical requirements for his or her sport. Dynamic balance is integral to most sports and can be assessed reliably using the star excursion or Y balance test, although these tests should not be used interchangeably.[4] Many sports necessitate high levels of functional loading, including single-leg force production and reduction. Athletes should therefore be competent during single-leg squatting, lateral hopping, and countermovement jumping. The absence of pain and compensatory strategies should be assessed throughout the movements. Excessive effort (eg, grimacing), loss of balance, loss of lumbopelvic control or knee alignment, or excessive trunk leaning generally indicate that the athlete is not ready to produce or control heavy impact or deceleration forces. Depending on the sport, single-leg loading can be modified to include endurance, multidirectional, or cognitive challenges.

Running form should be symmetrical and should not change significantly with fatigue. It is therefore important that athletes be challenged at running intensities that align with the specific energy demands of their sport (aerobic, anaerobic, mixed-energy system). Where applicable, athletes should be comfortable with the addition of multidirectional movements, task-specific agility, sport-specific skills, or unanticipated movement. In all cases, there should be no significant posttest response such as reactive swelling, increased pain, or any signs of anxiety or apprehension.

Conclusion

Although we have focused primarily on functional criteria, we should be cognizant that many additional factors (such as patient demographics, injury history, limb dominance, type of sport [contact, noncontact, collision], playing position, potential for taping, level of competition, stage of season, or fear of litigation) can influence the convalescence period after ankle sprain and the level of risk associated with our return-to-sport decisions. Determining readiness to return to sport after injury is often challenging. By highlighting sport-specific criteria and functional goals, we can facilitate a safer transition back to sport after ankle sprain. Meeting each criterion often requires a recursive approach that is facilitated through a tailored, stepwise approach to rehabilitation.

References

1. Doherty C, Delahunt E, Caulfield B, et al. The incidence and prevalence of ankle sprain injury: a systematic review and meta-analysis of prospective epidemiological studies. *Sports Med.* 2014;44:123-140.
2. Van Rijn RM, van Os AG, Bernsen RMD, et al. What is the clinical course of acute ankle sprains? A systematic literature review. *Am J Med.* 2008;121:324-331.
3. Herrington L, Myer G, Horsley I. Task based rehabilitation protocol for elite athletes following anterior cruciate ligament reconstruction: a clinical commentary. *Phys Ther Sport.* 2013;14:188-198.
4. Coughlan GF, Fullam K, Delahunt E, Gissane C, Caulfield BM. A comparison between performance on selected directions of the star excursion balance test and the Y balance test. *J Athl Train.* 2012;47:366-371.

HOW EFFECTIVE ARE FOOT ORTHOTICS IN TREATING IMPAIRMENTS ASSOCIATED WITH ANKLE SPRAINS?

Caitlin Whale, MS, LAT, ATC and
Carl G. Mattacola, PhD, ATC, FNATA

Ankle sprains are one of the most common injuries, with patients presenting with short-term impairments and a risk of long-term impairments. Several risk factors have been associated with ankle sprains, yet intervention strategies for preventing or treating them are varied. Postural control deficits,[1-3] pain,[1] limited range of motion, and muscular impairments are present following an ankle sprain. It is theorized that the sensory receptors located in the skin, muscles, and ligaments are disrupted, resulting in a deficit in the information provided to the central nervous system. The level of deficit after injury is of concern, because the level of impairment can have an effect on the functional recovery, possibly preventing a full recovery. Thus, interventions should address both the sensory and neuromuscular (motor) components of the injury.

Clinicians have the opportunity to choose between a wide variety of interventions to treat impairments after an acute ankle sprain. Ankle orthoses (ie, braces), surround the ankle joint and control motion at both the subtalar joint and the talocrural joint. Ankle orthoses provide effective stability but can be cumbersome and bulky. Orthotic intervention is an adjunct therapy for treating malalignments of the foot. Orthotics are created from the mold of a negative impression of the foot

McKeon PO, Wikstrom E, eds. *Quick Questions in
Ankle Sprains: Expert Advice in Sports Medicine* (pp 135-138).
© 2015 SLACK Incorporated.

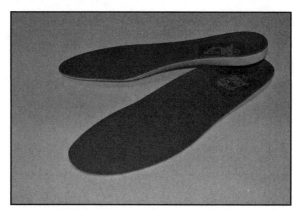

Figure 26-1. Ortho Arch® sport model semirigid orthotics. (Reprinted with permission from Foot Management, Inc.)

in a subtalar neutral position. From the mold, a soft, semirigid, or rigid orthotic can be manufactured. Orthotics are prescribed to aid in the realignment of the foot to a neutral position. A neutral position theoretically decreases the potential for injury and overuse by providing a more efficient foot position to maximize muscular efficiency. A neutral position is defined as the position in which the talus is equidistant within the mortise and is often depicted as a position in which the midline of the distal one-third of the lower leg and the midline of the calcaneus vertical. Additionally, realigning the foot to a neutral position may provide an advantage when maintaining balance. Improvement in postural stability for unimpaired individuals and for individuals with rearfoot malalignment during an orthotic condition has been reported.[4]

Orthotic interventions (Figure 26-1) have been investigated as a possible treatment option for both pain and sensorimotor impairments following an ankle sprain. The preservation of a neutral position with the application of orthotics reduces the stress on the injured structures by preventing excessive movement. It has been documented that individuals who have sustained an acute ankle sprain have greater postural sway, measured via a balance task, than do healthy individuals,[2,3] and the application of orthotics resulted in improved postural sway.[1,2] More specifically, an eyes-open, single-limb stance measured as time out of balance[1] and distance translated from the center of balance[2] have been reported to be improved following orthotic intervention. In addition, single-limb, eyes-closed postural sway was improved in both a group with calcaneal malalignment and an unimpaired control group who were treated with custom-molded orthotics.[4] It is theorized that the improvements in postural sway are due to increased somatosensory afferent input from the orthotics.[4] The increased surface area between the orthotic and the foot increases pressure against the sole of the foot and stimulates mechanoreceptors that are sensitive to changes in pressure, thereby increasing somatosensory feedback to the central nervous system. The application of custom-molded orthotics has also been shown to significantly reduce pain during a jogging task in individuals who sustained a lateral ankle sprain when compared to healthy individuals.[1]

While it appears that there may be a functional benefit to the use of foot orthotics following ankle sprains, evidence supporting their use is not conclusive. In a study in which the performance of several different orthoses was compared to the use of no orthotics, none of the orthotic conditions improved postural control over that of the control condition (no orthotic at all).[3] The lack of a difference may be due to differences in the methodology utilized. A simple single-limb balance task on a stable surface was used to assess balance.[3] It is possible that the demands of balancing on a stable surface were not challenging, such that balance was compromised to an extent that orthotics would provide an advantage. When postural demands increased in dynamic balance conditions, the effects of the orthotics on postural control were more pronounced.[1,2] Therefore, the effectiveness of orthotics may be more detectable in a dynamic condition than in a static condition.

Chronic ankle instability (CAI) can be described as recurrent instability or feeling of giving way coupled with lingering symptoms. Many of the impairments associated with CAI are apparent during dynamic balance activities and are similar to the impairments associated with ankle sprains. Specifically, individuals with CAI often have diminished postural control and use compensatory strategies to maintain balance. The addition of an orthotic intervention provides continual somatosensory feedback because of the pressure the orthotic exerts on the plantar surface of the foot. This increase in somatosensory feedback may aid in individuals' ability to maintain a stable base of support. Although the evidence is limited, the use of orthotics with CAI may be beneficial during dynamic conditions.[5] During a 4-week orthotic intervention, participants with CAI demonstrated improvements in the medial, anterolateral, and posterolateral directions of the star excursion balance test.[5] The positive results presented here are promising; however, to fully understand the effect of orthotics in individuals with CAI, further research should be conducted.

To date, there is no clear consensus on the most appropriate intervention strategy for treating impairments after ankle sprains; however, orthotics should be given consideration as an effective adjunct. On the basis of the literature, orthotic interventions are effective in improving postural sway and pain after ankle sprains[1,2] and dynamic balance impairments in those with CAI.[5] Therefore, while in the acute phase (3 to 6 weeks) of an ankle sprain, it is recommended that custom-molded orthotics be implemented in the treatment of postural instability deficits and pain during activity. Furthermore, in individuals with CAI, custom-molded orthotics are recommended for improvements in dynamic balance impairments, but their effectiveness for injury prevention or for reducing the incidence of sprains is not supported and needs further study.

References

1. Orteza LC, Vogelbach WD, Denegar CR. The effect of molded and unmolded orthotics on balance and pain while jogging following inversion ankle sprain. *J Athl Train*. 1992;27:80.
2. Guskiewicz KM, Perrin D. Effect of orthotics on postural sway following inversion ankle sprain. *J Orthop Sports Phys Ther*. 1996;23:326-331.
3. Hertel J, Denegar CR, Buckley W, Sharkey NA, Stokes WL. Effect of rearfoot orthotics on postural sway after lateral ankle sprain. *Arch Phys Med Rehabil*. 2001;82:1000-1003.
4. Mattacola CG, Dwyer MK, Miller AK, et al. Effect of orthoses on postural stability in asymptomatic subjects with rearfoot malalignment during a 6-week acclimation period. *Arch Phys Med Rehabil*. 2007;88:653-660.
5. Sesma AR, Mattacola CG, Uhl TL, Nitz AJ, McKeon PO. Effect of foot orthotics on single- and double-limb dynamic balance tasks in patients with chronic ankle instability. *Foot Ankle Spec*. 2008;1:330-337.

TO WHAT EXTENT DOES INTRINSIC FOOT MUSCLE STRENGTHENING ENHANCE REHABILITATION OUTCOMES FOR ANKLE SPRAINS?

François Fourchet, PT, PhD; Darren James, PhD; and Patrick O. McKeon, PhD, ATC, CSCS

The primary objective for the health care provider in rehabilitating a patient following a lateral ankle sprain is the restoration of full ankle joint range of motion and neuromuscular coordination to the preinjury state. It is known that 85% of all ankle sprains occur in the lateral ligaments of the ankle, and reinjury rates are known to be as high as 70% in certain sporting populations. Such recurrence is termed *chronic ankle instability* and is believed to be a combination of mechanical and functional factors. A very important consideration for ankle sprains is that no muscles directly attach to the talus, which means that all the dynamic stability of both the subtalar and talocrural joints comes from contributions of muscles that attach or originate in bones above or below these joints. Functional instability of the ankle joint is defined in sufferers who experience one or more of the following: impaired postural control, neuromuscular deficits, proprioceptive deficits, and strength deficits.

Currently, all foot and ankle exercises prescribed by the American Academy of Orthopaedic Surgeons (http://orthoinfo.aaos.org/topic.cfm?topic=a00150) during

McKeon PO, Wikstrom EA, eds. *Quick Questions in Ankle Sprains: Expert Advice in Sports Medicine* (pp 139-142).

phase 2 of rehabilitation from grade 1 and 2 ankle sprains essentially target the extrinsic foot muscles (EFMs) to help the athlete regain an adequate level of ankle joint stability. The premise for this rationale is that all of these muscles cross the ankle joints and therefore may enhance the dynamic control of the ankle. However, on the basis of the high recurrence rate of ankle sprains, it appears that these rehabilitation recommendations may be inadequate. A group of muscles that have received far less attention in the literature on ankle sprain rehabilitation are the intrinsic foot muscles (IFMs): those muscles that both originate and insert in the foot. These muscles are much smaller than their EFM counterparts but may play a much different and necessary role in proper foot function.[1] The functional relationship of the IFMs and EFMs has led to the theory that these muscles function as a core system, similar to the lumbopelvic core system.[1] The IFMs function as the local stabilizers of the foot, whereas the EFMs function as the global movers. On the basis of their electromyographic activation profiles, the IFMs function to stabilize the foot-ankle complex during single-limb stance and propulsion during walking and running. Because the IFMs are most commonly neglected in the ankle sprain rehabilitation process, an essential element of foot core stability is not addressed. The purpose of this chapter is to provide a guide for incorporating foot core training in ankle sprain rehabilitation.

One of the key exercises in foot core training is the "short foot exercise."[1] In this exercise, the patient is asked to contract the IFMs in an isolated manner to raise the medial longitudinal arch. This technique is akin to the abdominal draw-in maneuver during lumbopelvic core training. As the patient learns to activate the IFMs through the short foot exercise in a seated position, the demands of the exercise are gradually progressed to more challenging activities in double- and single-limb standing and landing. Four weeks of short foot exercise training has been shown to improve both local foot postural control (maintaining an arch during standing activities) and dynamic single-leg balance. Also, short foot exercise training has been shown to enhance self-reported function in patients with chronic ankle instability.[2] Training the IFMs appears to be an important component for a foot and ankle rehabilitation program, but a major challenge for clinicians is getting patients to understand how to isolate and activate them. Proper instruction in the short foot exercise technique is essential for its success, but many patients struggle to isolate these muscles.

A complimentary modality for the short foot exercise is neuromuscular electrical stimulation (NMES) of the IFM, which appears promising as a tool in rehabilitation. In essence, this approach can be used to educate patients during the initial stages of rehabilitation by allowing them to understand the precise biomechanics of foot function with involuntary activation of the IFMs rather than trying to have them figure out how to activate these muscles voluntarily. NMES has been

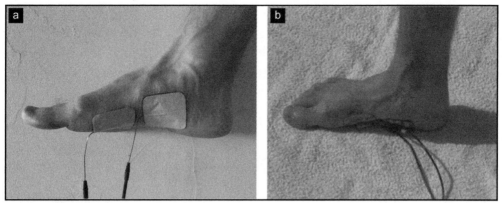

Figure 27-1. Localization of the electrodes under the medial longitudinal arch of the foot (a)[4-6] and at the AH level (b).[3] (Figure 27-1a from Fourchet F, Kilgallon M, Loepelt H, Millet GP. Plantar muscles electro-stimulation and navicular drop. *Sci Sports.* 2009;24:262-264. Copyright © 2009 Elsevier Masson SAS. All rights reserved.)

reported to increase neural activation, and strengthen human skeletal muscle, complement voluntary exercise and has been posited as a rehabilitative tool for pathologies that compromise normal neuromuscular function.[3] The incorporation of an NMES protocol on the IFMs with muscle strengthening over several weeks of IFM training has been shown to enhance foot postural control and plantar pressure profiles during running.[4,5]

In both cases, we found promising results confirming that NMES to the medial longitudinal arch (Figure 27-1) had an effect as it prevented arch collapse and hyperpronation in dynamic conditions. It is apparent that this type of training has an impact on the foot core system. Positive results were also observed when NMES was delivered to a specific IFM, namely the abductor hallucis (AH).[3,6] This muscle's activation profile is regarded as a surrogate for all medially located IFMs; moreover, it has the largest cross-sectional area and is the strongest muscle within the foot.[1] After only a 20-minute session of NMES, significant alterations in plantar pressure distribution were observed while subjects maintained a static stance position.[6] These results (greater rear-foot inversion and a higher arch) led Gaillet et al[6] to conclude that enhanced balance control is associated with AH stimulation. On the basis of these results and those from short foot exercise training, the incorporation of NMES with short foot exercises to restore proper foot core strength should be considered when designing rehabilitation programs after ankle sprain.[1] A logical shift from NMES to voluntary activation of the IFMs during rehabilitation progression is also recommended.

From the evidence presented in this chapter, it is important to consider foot core training in ankle sprain rehabilitation. The incorporation of NMES can help to educate patients about proper activation of the IFMs if they are unfamiliar with the short foot exercise or these muscles have been inhibited due to injury. Central to its inclusion as a complementary technique is the reported "neural" effect with use, which is in essence the primary objective in rehabilitation following a lateral ankle sprain. Restoring the dynamic nature of the foot is critically important for enhancing the ability to cope with changing environmental and task demands and may be a missing link in the rehabilitation of ankle injuries.

References

1. McKeon PO, Hertel J, Bramble D, Davis I. The foot core system: a new paradigm for understanding intrinsic foot muscle function. *Br J Sports Med.*
2. Drewes LK. Effects of rehabilitation incorporating short foot exercises on functional outcomes for chronic ankle instability [doctoral dissertation]. Charlottesville, VA: Human Services, University of Virginia; 2009.
3. James DC, Chesters T, Sumners DP, et al. Wide-pulse electrical stimulation to an intrinsic foot muscle induces acute functional changes in forefoot-rearfoot coupling behaviour during walking. *Int J Sports Med.* 2013;34:438-443.
4. Fourchet F, Kuitunen S, Girard O, Beard AJ, Millet GP. Effects of combined foot/ankle electromyostimulation and resistance training on the in-shoe plantar pressure patterns during sprint in young athletes. *J Sports Sci Med.* 2011;10:292-300.
5. Fourchet F, Kilgallon M, Loepelt H, Millet GP. Plantar muscles electro-stimulation and navicular drop. *Sci Sports.* 2009;24:262-264.
6. Gaillet JC, Biraud JC, Bessou M, Bessou P. Modifications of baropodograms after transcutaneous electric stimulation of the abductor hallucis muscle in humans standing erect. *Clin Biomech (Bristol, Avon).* 2004;19:1066-1069.

How Should I Design a Rehabilitation Program for Chronic Ankle Instability, and How Long Should It Last?

Eric Eils, Prof. Dr. rer. medic. habil.

Chronic ankle instability (CAI) refers to the occurrence of persistent symptoms after initial ankle sprain(s), although athletes or patients may have returned to full activity. These persistent symptoms may include repeated inversion sprains, pain, and loss of function or a subjective feeling of the ankle giving way. A mechanical or functional instability or a combination of both is thought to be the cause of CAI. Mechanical instability describes the entity of mechanical impairments to the ankle joint (eg, pathologic laxity of the ligaments), whereas functional instability refers to neuromuscular alterations (eg, loss of control or proprioceptive deficits).

These deficits may be evaluated using specific test methods. It has been shown that athletes suffering from CAI have mechanical or functional deficits such as increased laxity of ankle ligaments or diminished joint position sense as indicated in impaired ankle reproduction capabilities, respectively. However, a combination of both mechanical and functional instability is also possible, and one entity does not necessarily imply the existence of the other, which makes it more difficult to adequately diagnose deficits in properties or function. These aspects underline the fact that not all cases of CAI are alike; therefore, different aspects should be considered when rehabilitation is addressed appropriately.

McKeon PO, Wikstrom EA, eds. *Quick Questions in Ankle Sprains: Expert Advice in Sports Medicine* (pp 143-148).

Different models have been developed to better understand the potential contributing factors to CAI and their interdependence. Although these models provide a basis for understanding these factors, they fail to link specific deficits of athletes to suitable intervention methods. Recently, an approach was taken to address specific deficits to interventions subdivided into domains such as range of motion, strength, balance, and functional activities.[1] With the help of this specific approach and the theoretical basis of the provided models, it seems possible to selectively influence the rehabilitation process by using specific measured deficits.

However, neuromuscular training (ie, programs that include proprioceptive, strength, or postural stability exercises) and rehabilitation programs are often not designed as a result of evaluated deficits but are selected from the literature regarding programs that previously proved successful. On the one hand, this appears problematic, given the fact that several of these existing programs differ extensively in design and dose-response relationship (eg, several times per week training on an ankle disk to a multistation circuit training once per week). Besides that, there is no consensus on integration or elimination of further sensory systems (visual, vestibular, somatosensory), implementation methods (eg, duration, intensity, density), specific design of exercises, or organizational considerations (training on a separate basis or included within normal training routines, timing of training within one training routine). On the other hand, it is sometimes impossible to specifically address athletes' requirements due to organizational considerations, as in team sports or groups in which different players with different deficits must be trained simultaneously.

There seem to be 2 lines of research for CAI: changes in outcome measures in response to rehabilitation (balance, proprioception, etc) and evaluation of the recurrence of injury after rehabilitation. However, there is a lack of evidence that links the two.[2]

Recently, a new paradigm for the rehabilitation of patients with CAI was proposed that combined patient-specific deficits with appropriate interventions.[1] This is actually a promising advance, because most other programs are more general and do not focus on individual deficits.[2,3] However, those general proprioceptive programs are successful in the prevention and rehabilitation of ankle sprains with an emphasis on CAI. In general, precise identification of deficits and a specifically designed rehabilitation program may be more effective than generic programs in the treatment of single patients suffering from CAI. As mentioned earlier, an integration of such programs within a normal training routine of, for example, basketball players is often hard to achieve because of organizational factors or the simple fact that not all patients with CAI are alike and not all players are suffering from CAI. The use of more general training routines with several different exercises and an increase or modification in difficulty levels is less specific (individually) but most probably successful, too. Therefore, these programs are also recommended for rehabilitation in patients with CAI.

Recommendations for the Design of Rehabilitation Programs in Patients or Athletes Suffering From Chronic Ankle Instability

In the following list, the most important aspects for the design of rehabilitation programs concerning CAI are highlighted in the context of earlier statements.

- Successful training interventions in the literature involved individuals aged 20 to 30 years. It seems safe to assume that training interventions are also applicable for older athlete populations. In this context, exercises should be modified accordingly.

- As a first step, individual deficits in athletes should be evaluated using different test procedures, and specific exercises should be derived. For example, if postural balance in a single-limb stance is impaired, specific one-leg exercises should be done.

- Training programs that address several aspects of neuromuscular control with variable exercises should be used if the evaluation of individual deficits is not possible. At this point, multistation programs in a circuit design are recommended.

- Training parameters
  - Absolute duration: The training period should last from a minimum of 4 to 6 weeks up to several months. This duration also depends on training intensity per week.
  - Intensity per week: Positive effects have been described in programs that were performed once per week and for 9 months, as well as for programs that were performed once or several times per week for 4 to 6 weeks. The intensity also depends on the absolute training duration. The exact dose-effect relationship remains unclear and still needs to be established.
  - Density (ratio of exercise/rest): Most exercise programs were performed for 30 to 45 seconds (one leg) followed by a 30-second break.
  - Time: When the training program is embedded within normal training routines, the athlete should be in a well-rested condition. It is conceivable that

exercises may be performed under controlled tiring conditions according to the actual status of patients/athletes.

○ Difficulty level: A progression in difficulty level should be apparent, and it should be adjusted accordingly. However, there is hardly any information available about the exact timing regarding when to advance to the next higher level.[4] This decision should depend on the individual performance of athletes. It should be considered that the focus of such neuromuscular training regimens is not to simply perform but also to sense. Some dual tasks such as catching and throwing balls might be added to preserve motivation and to adjust exercises to be more applied.

- Exercises should be performed while barefoot to diminish bracing effects of the shoes and to improve proprioceptive feedback.

- The input of different sensory systems should be impaired or modified. For example, visual information should be disabled by closing the eyes to lower the dominant role of the visual system in movement execution and to emphasize sensory information from periphery. Additional aids such as different pads, surfaces, or instability devices should be used in this context, too.

- Basic guiding principles from simple to more complex or from easier to harder should be followed.

Finally, Figure 28-1 illustrates some exercises especially designed for basketball, and a more detailed description of single exercises with related difficulty levels is provided in Table 28-1.

References

1. Donovan L, Hertel J. A new paradigm for rehabilitation of patients with chronic ankle instability. *Phys Sportsmed.* 2012;40:41-51.
2. Eils E, Schröter R, Schröder M, Gerss J, Rosenbaum D. Multistation proprioceptive exercise program prevents ankle injuries in basketball. *Med Sci Sports Exerc.* 2010;42:2098-2105.
3. Verhagen E, van der Beek A, Twisk J, et al. The effect of a proprioceptive balance board training program for the prevention of ankle sprains: a prospective controlled trial. *Am J Sports Med.* 2004;32:1385-1393.
4. Wikstrom EA, Hubbard-Turner T, McKeon PO. Understanding and treating lateral ankle sprains and their consequences: a constraints-based approach. *Sports Med.* 2013;43:385-393.

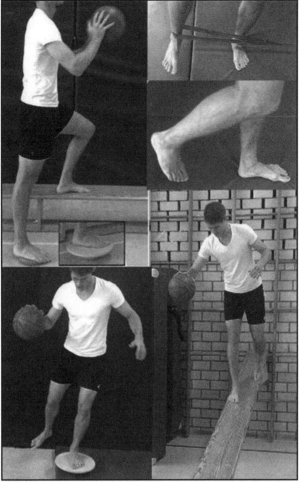

Figure 28-1. Examples of typical neuromuscular exercises. Some of these are especially adapted to basketball.

Table 28-1

Description of Single Exercises With Related Difficulty Levels

Sample Exercise	Basic	Variation 1	Variation 2
Unstable devices	Maintain balance in single-limb stance on air squab or ankle disk. The contralateral leg is rested on an inclined surface just partly being loaded.	Maintain balance in single-limb stance on air squab or ankle disk using a ball. Pass the ball to a partner or against a wall and regulate stance after catching the ball.	Maintain balance in single-limb stance on air squab or ankle disk. The contralateral leg is nearly elevated without being loaded. Further variation: Pass the ball to a partner or against a wall and regulate stance after catching the ball.
Ankle disk	Single-limb stance on an ankle disk. Stability of the ankle disk may be modified by using a piece of carpet or a mat underneath the device.	Single-limb stance on an ankle disk with eyes closed.	Single-limb stance on an ankle disk with open eyes and performing an additional task like catching and throwing a ball.
Uneven walkway	Walk on uneven walkway on different materials. Cover material with a blanket.	Change material to increase instability level.	Walk with closed eyes on material.
Elastic bands	Maintain balance in single-limb stance-elevating the contralateral leg against resistance of an elastic bandage.	Maintain balance in single-limb stance (eyes closed) elevating the contralateral leg against resistance of an elastic bandage.	Maintain balance in single-limb stance while moving the contralateral leg sideways against resistance of an elastic bandage. Evert the lateral border of the contralateral leg.

WHAT IS THE ROLE OF PROXIMAL STRENGTH AND NEUROMUSCULAR TRAINING IN ANKLE REHABILITATION?

Phillip Gribble, PhD, ATC, FNATA and
Masafumi Terada, PhD, ATC

Deficits in range of motion (ROM), strength, neuromuscular (NM) control, and balance are typically present in patients with acute ankle sprains. Most of these disabilities persist in those with chronic ankle instability (CAI) as well. Therefore, traditional rehabilitation for ankle sprains and CAI consists of interventions to restore ROM, strength, and NM control at the ankle and to restore balance and functional movement performance.[1] While these protocols are usually effective at treating impairments at the ankle and overcoming disability, the high rates of ankle sprain recurrence and development of CAI already discussed in the previous questions raise the need to critique the effectiveness of traditional ankle rehabilitation to address all impairments that may exist.

Similar impairments in strength and NM control may also present in areas proximal to the ankle. We cannot present a thorough review of the literature in this context, but the evidence is growing that alterations and deficits in strength and NM control at the knee, the hip, and the trunk are associated with facets of ankle instability. Why these changes occur remains unknown, but one theory involves changes in spinal and supraspinal pathways that may persist in patients with CAI.[2] The information to date has only been observed in retrospective study designs,

McKeon PO, Wikstrom EA, eds. *Quick Questions in
Ankle Sprains: Expert Advice in Sports Medicine* (pp 149-153).
© 2015 SLACK Incorporated.

so it is as yet unknown if these alterations cause or are the effect of ankle injury. Nonetheless, the presence of these changes in knee, hip, and trunk function in patients with CAI suggests the possibility for evaluating more than just the ankle to determine avenues for improvement.

The literature includes a plethora of examples of strength and NM control deficits in patients with ankle injury, both acute and chronic. While the volume of information is not the same, there is a growing body of work that shows deficits in strength throughout the lower limbs in these patient populations. For example, Gribble and Robinson[3] reported an ankle and knee strength deficit in patients with unilateral CAI. Using isokinetic testing, patients with CAI not only had ankle plantar flexion force production deficits but also demonstrated deficits in knee flexion and extension force production.

Altered muscle-activation patterns have been observed in the ankles of patients with ankle instability, but there is also an abundance of literature suggesting similar altered patterns in muscles controlling the knee, the hip, and the trunk in these populations. A recent example of this was demonstrated in the gluteal muscles during multiple tasks reliant on hip movement.[4] Patients with CAI demonstrated a reduced peak gluteal muscle activation, especially the gluteus maximus, during single-plane and multiple-plane movements, compared to participants with no history of ankle sprain. Implementing exercises that can highly activate hip muscles may be considered in clinical interventions for CAI to restore NM control and strength at the hip, although future intervention studies are necessary. An example of the hip movements can be seen in Figure 29-1.

Neuromuscular control can also be described by movement patterns using kinematic assessments during a variety of tasks. Examples of altered patterns of foot position in patients with ankle instability during gait and landing can be found throughout the literature. The placement of the ankle complex in space to make proper ground contact depends on proper control of the joints proximal to the ankle. Therefore, examining the movement patterns of the knee and hip during functional tasks may provide insight into the placement of the ankle that may create injurious mechanisms. At this point, there is limited, but consistent, information that suggests that altered movement patterns of the knee and hip exist in patients with CAI. For instance, altered knee flexion patterns exist during landing in patients with CAI, which help to explain overall decreased dynamic stability.[5] Educating patients with CAI with regard to proper mechanics at the proximal joints in the lower extremity during functional activities, such as increasing knee flexion angle during jump landing, may be addressed in clinical interventions for patients with CAI.

Deficits and alterations in the joints proximal to the ankle in patients with CAI have been quantified but largely ignored when it comes to developing prevention

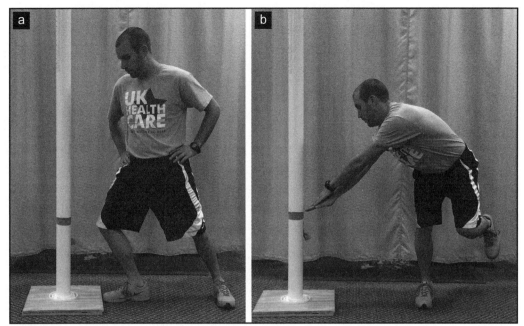

Figure 29-1. Hip functional movements that can be used to detect deficits in CAI gluteal muscle activation[4]: (A) rotational lunge; (B) rotational squat.

and rehabilitation protocols. However, we are aware of no published data that incorporate interventions to the knee, hip, and trunk complexes in patients with CAI. However, pilot data from our laboratory group show the potential for success using this approach. Using a randomized control trial design, we completed a 6-week intervention study to determine the effectiveness of a proximal joint exercise protocol at improving self-reported disability and dynamic stability in patients with CAI. Patients with unilateral CAI were randomly assigned to a group that performed "traditional" ankle rehabilitation (AR) exercises (Thera-Band ankle resistance movements, wobbleboard, single-limb balance), a group that performed proximal joint-focused rehabilitation (PR) exercises (straight-leg raises, knee flexion/extension resistance movements, single-leg squats), or a control/no-exercise group. We assessed the effectiveness of these therapeutic exercise protocols using the foot and ankle disability index (FADI) activities of daily living and sports scales to represent a patient-generated outcome measure of self-reported ankle disability and also a clinically oriented outcome measure called the resultant vector time to stabilization (RVTTS), which represented dynamic stability during a single-leg landing task. The outcomes from this unpublished study can be found in Figure 29-2.

The AR and PR groups improved in all 3 measures (FADI and FADI-sport showed increased scores and RVTTS had decreased time) compared to the control group, but the PR group also had significant improvements in these outcomes

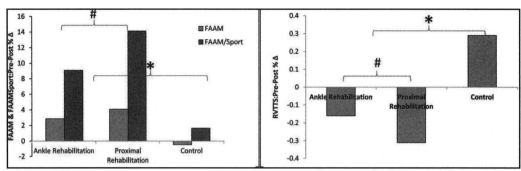

Figure 29-2. Comparison of changes in self-reported disability and dynamic stability in patients with CAI who underwent ankle rehabilitation (AR), proximal joint rehabilitation (PR), or no intervention (control). *AR and PR > control (p < .05). #PR > AR (p < .05). FAAM = foot and ankle ability measure. (Gribble and Shinohara, unpublished data).

compared to the AR group. This suggests that AR is effective at improving outcomes in patients with CAI, but the introduction of PR protocols may provide additional benefits that clinicians should begin considering. We advocate for the continued investigation of this relationship using clinical trials to determine what interventions can address NM control alterations and deficits throughout the kinetic chain, especially in the joints proximal to the ankle.

Conclusion

Altered NM control, including strength, activation, and movement patterns, exist in the knee, hip, and trunk in patients with CAI and is likely an illustration of central nervous system changes. While the information that defines these altered relationships is present, the application into intervention is promising but needs further investigation. Additionally, the information that does exist on deficits in knee and hip NM control has been gained from retrospective study designs, making it difficult to know if patients with ankle instability develop adaptations to proximal joints following injury or if these phenomena may exist inherently and may help to explain ankle injury and the development of CAI. For now, clinicians should consider evaluating the NM control throughout the lower extremity of patients who present with ankle instability and determine how best to incorporate intervention to address these findings.

References

1. O'Driscoll J, Delahunt E. Neuromuscular training to enhance sensorimotor and functional deficits in subjects with chronic ankle instability: a systematic review and best evidence synthesis. *Sports Med Arthrosc Rehabil Ther & Technol.* 2011;3:19.
2. Hass CJ, Bishop MD, Doidge D, Wikstrom EA. Chronic ankle instability alters central organization of movement. *Am J Sports Med.* 2010;38:829-834.
3. Gribble P, Robinson R. An examination of ankle, knee, and hip torque production in individuals with chronic ankle instability. *J Strength Cond Res.* 2009;23:395-400.
4. Webster KA, Gribble PA. A comparison of electromyography of gluteus medius and maximus in subjects with and without chronic ankle instability during two functional exercises. *Phys Ther Sport.* 2013;14:17-22.
5. Gribble P, Robinson R. Differences in spatiotemporal landing variables during a dynamic stability task in subjects with CAI. *Scand J Med Sci Sports.* 2010;20:e63-e71.

To What Extent Should I Use Manipulative Therapies to Treat Ankle Sprains and Chronic Ankle Instability?

Matthew C. Hoch, PhD, ATC and
Bill Vicenzino, PhD

Decreases in ankle dorsiflexion range of motion are frequently identified in patients with a history of ankle sprain or chronic ankle instability. In these patients, dorsiflexion range-of-motion deficits have been linked to changes in motion and positioning of the talus and fibula relative to the ankle mortise or tibia. Specifically, individuals who have sustained an ankle sprain are more likely to exhibit restrictions in posterior talar glide, and individuals with chronic ankle instability are more likely to have an anterior positional fault of the talus or distal fibula.[1-3] Cumulatively, these deficits suggest that the basis for decreased dorsiflexion following ankle injury is alterations in motion and position of the articulating surfaces within the joint. Dorsiflexion impairments often are accompanied by other deleterious symptoms and impairments following ankle injury, such as pain, diminished sensorimotor function, activity limitations, and participation restrictions. Therefore, dorsiflexion range-of-motion deficits are common in individuals with a history of ankle sprain and may have implications on recovery following an ankle sprain and the progression to chronic ankle instability.

Several manual therapy interventions for restoring mechanical ankle function, reducing pain, and increasing function in patients with ankle sprain and

McKeon PO, Wikstrom EA, eds. *Quick Questions in Ankle Sprains: Expert Advice in Sports Medicine* (pp 155-159).
© 2015 SLACK Incorporated.

individuals with chronic ankle instability have been examined (Table 30-1). Most of these interventions involve joint mobilization or manipulation techniques that focus on restoring normal positioning and movement of the talus or distal fibula by passively gliding these structures posteriorly to increase dorsiflexion range of motion. Beyond the mechanical benefits of restoring motion within a joint, several investigators have found that there are neurophysiological benefits of joint mobilization and manipulation as well as enhanced patient-reported outcomes such as improvements in activity limitations and participation restrictions. This suggests that the basis by which manual therapies are used to treat ankle sprains and chronic ankle instability should be considered from mechanical, neurophysiological, and patient-centered perspectives.

For patients with an ankle sprain and chronic ankle instability, the treatment goals for manual therapy are typically associated with increasing dorsiflexion range of motion, reducing pain or improving sensorimotor function, and improving patient-reported function. A recent systematic review evaluated all of the randomized controlled trials that have examined the effectiveness of joint mobilization or manipulation in the treatment of lateral ankle sprains.[4] Eight studies that used a range of manual therapy interventions, including anterior-to-posterior talar glides, talocrural distraction, talocrural mobilization-with-movement, and talocrural manipulation, were included. On the basis of the included studies, there is strong evidence that these manual therapy interventions were successful at diminishing pain and increasing dorsiflexion range of motion in patients with acute ankle sprain. A literature review was also conducted to synthesize the studies that examined the effectiveness of joint mobilization or manipulation in the treatment of chronic ankle instability.[3] The studies included in this review examined several manual therapy interventions, which included anterior-to-posterior talar glides, distal fibular manipulation, and talocrural mobilization with movement. All of the included studies that directed treatment at the talocrural joint were able to increase dorsiflexion range of motion. From a neurophysiological perspective, there was evidence that manual therapies can transiently improve certain aspects of sensorimotor function including single-limb balance, ankle joint position sense, and muscle activation. Since the time of the literature review,[3] one additional study examined the effects of multiple talocrural mobilization-with-movement treatments.[5] No improvements in dorsiflexion range of motion or single-limb balance were detected after treatment, but improvements were detected in sports-related patient-reported function. Across both reviews of the evidence,[3,4] there was a limited amount of patient-centered evidence indicating that very few studies have examined changes in activity and participation from the patient's point of view. Additionally, a major limitation identified in both reviews[3,4] was the lack of long-term follow-up,

<u>Table 30-1</u>

Manual Therapy Interventions to Restore Mechanical Ankle Function, Reduce Pain, and Increase Function in Ankle Sprain Patients and Individuals With Chronic Ankle Instability

Technique	Description
Talocrural anterior-to-posterior mobilization/manipulation[3,4]	The patient is positioned supine with the foot suspended off the treatment plinth.
	The clinician stabilizes the distal tibia and fibula with one hand and applies an anterior-to-posterior glide of the talus with the opposite hand.
	The rate of oscillation, oscillation amplitude, and additional treatment parameters are dictated by the patient presentation and treatment goals.
Talocrural weight-bearing posterior-to-anterior mobilization[3,5]	The patient is positioned in a kneeling lunge position on a treatment plinth with the involved limb in a weight-bearing stance and the foot in a neutral position.
	A nonelastic nylon belt is placed around the distal aspect of the tibia and fibula and around the waist of the clinician.
	The clinician stabilizes the talus and forefoot by applying pressure on the talus and forefoot followed by a posterior-to-anterior glide of the tibia over the talus using the belt.
	The clinician continues applying pressure as the participant moves into dorsiflexion until discomfort is reported or the end range of motion occurs.
Distal tibiofibular mobilization/manipulation[3]	The patient is positioned supine with the foot suspended off the treatment plinth.
	The clinician stabilizes the distal tibia with one hand while grasping the distal fibula between the fingers and the thenar eminence while creating an anterior-to-posterior glide with the opposite hand.
	The rate of oscillation, oscillation amplitude, and additional treatment parameters are dictated by the patient presentation and treatment goals.

(continued)

Table 30-1 (continued)

Manual Therapy Interventions to Restore Mechanical Ankle Function, Reduce Pain, and Increase Function in Ankle Sprain Patients and Individuals With Chronic Ankle Instability

Talocrural distraction[3,4]	The patient is positioned supine with the foot suspended off the treatment plinth.
	The clinician positions the fingers of both hands over the dorsum of the foot and the thumbs over the plantar surface of the foot.
	Force is applied to distract the talus distally from the ankle mortise.
	The rate, amplitude, and volume of distraction are dictated by the patient presentation and treatment goals.

which limits the ability to make conclusions regarding the long-term effects of these treatments.

Overall, the extent to which manual therapies should be used to treat ankle sprains and chronic ankle instability depends on the patient-centered need to have increased dorsiflexion and reduced pain. While there is some limited support that manual therapies can benefit sensorimotor function and improve patient-reported function in individuals with chronic ankle instability, more studies using similar outcomes are required to make a clear recommendation. It is also uncertain if manual therapies can reduce the risk of recurrent injury, residual symptoms, or the development of chronic ankle instability due to the limited follow-up in the majority of studies. Manual therapy interventions may be effective, but the range of intervention techniques and outcomes that have been examined in the literature have yielded inconsistency in their benefits for those with ankle instability issues. The exact mechanisms underpinning the mechanical and neurophysiologic changes following manual therapies also need to be elucidated to determine which patients may benefit most from these treatments. Finally, it should be noted that no adverse or deleterious effects of manual therapy have been reported in the literature, which suggests that these techniques are likely not harmful when performed correctly in individuals with a history of ankle sprain. It is recommended that the research evidence be combined with clinician expertise and patient values when considering the extent to which manual therapies should be used in clinical practice. Combining the research evidence with the systematic documentation of patient outcomes and patient values will lead to more robust recommendations.

References

1. Denegar CR, Hertel J, Fonseca J. The effect of lateral ankle sprain on dorsiflexion range of motion, posterior talar glide, and joint laxity. *J Orthop Sport Phys Ther*. 2002;32:166-173.
2. Wikstrom EA, Hubbard TJ. Talar positional fault in persons with chronic ankle instability. *Arch Phys Med Rehabil*. 2010;91:1267-1271.
3. Hoch MC, Grindstaff TL. Effectiveness of joint mobilization in patients with chronic ankle instability. *Athl Train Sports Health Care*. 2012;4:237-244.
4. Loudon JK, Reiman MP, Sylvain J. The efficacy of manual joint mobilisation/manipulation in treatment of lateral ankle sprains: a systematic review. *Br J Sport Med*. 2014;48:365-370.
5. Gilbreath JP, Gaven SL, Van Lunen BL, Hoch MC. The effects of mobilization with movement on dorsiflexion range of motion, dynamic balance, and self-reported function in individuals with chronic ankle instability. *Man Ther*. 2014;19:152-157.

QUESTION **31**

WHAT PHYSICAL AND PHARMACOLOGICAL AGENTS ARE USEFUL WHEN TREATING ANKLE SPRAINS?

Chris M. Bleakley, PhD, BSc

Ankle sprains are one of the most common musculoskeletal injuries in sport, particularly those involving the lateral complex. A fundamental objective in the immediate stages after injury is to protect the joint to minimize bleeding and prevent excessive distension or rerupture at the injury site. As the injury progresses, protection should be replaced with a functional management approach. This involves progressive weight bearing and walking, which have been shown to be more effective than passive approaches such as immobilization and casting after mild or moderate ankle sprains.[1] This chapter provides an overview of various treatments that can be used effectively in conjunction with the functional management of ankle sprains.

Non steroidal anti-inflammatory drugs (NSAIDs) are perhaps the most commonly prescribed pharmacological agents for ankle sprains. NSAIDs work through cyclooxygenase inhibition, which blocks prostaglandin production and causes analgesic, anti-inflammatory, and antithrombotic effects. Evidence from randomized placebo-controlled trials shows that NSAIDs have a consistent analgesic effect after an ankle sprain.[2] However, a significant limitation is that these studies did not include long-term follow-up, and there is no evidence that they enhance

McKeon PO, Wikstrom EA, eds. *Quick Questions in Ankle Sprains: Expert Advice in Sports Medicine* (pp 161-164).

important functional outcomes. Recent consensus guidelines[2] support the use of NSAIDs after some acute musculoskeletal injuries; however, they advise judicious use after ankle sprains. An ongoing concern is that NSAIDs have a deleterious effect on mechanical stability, which could be a result of aggressive tissue loading due to their anesthetic effects or a direct biological impairment of ligament healing. There is a risk of significant adverse events with NSAIDs involving the gastrointestinal, renal, and cardiovascular systems; however, they are primarily associated with long-term use. NSAIDs may be most suitable for more complex ankle sprains in which the patient presents with concomitant joint synovitis.[2] For many ankle sprains, simple analgesic medications such as paracetamol/acetaminophen may provide a suitable alternative, particularly in the acute phases when reducing pain is the primary goal.

Cryotherapy is one of the most commonly used modalities in the management of acute soft-tissue injury. Topical ice application provides a significant analgesic effect and is one of the cheapest and most effective methods for enhancing patient comfort in the acute phases after ankle sprain. Cryotherapy offers additional therapeutic benefit when it is used in conjunction with therapeutic exercises. This approach is often referred to as cryokinetics, and it is particularly useful during the early stages of the rehabilitative process. Its primary effects include the (re)activation of ankle musculature and earlier restoration of normal functional movement patterns. Cryokinetics is most effective when the exercise content and dosage align with the stage of tissue healing.[3] Its key premise is to improve the quality of the therapeutic movement, and it is not appropriate to use cryotherapy to facilitate aggressive or fast-tracked rehabilitation.

Throughout recovery, rehabilitation exercises should continue to promote progressive mechanical loading on the ankle. This is essential not only for enhancing functional recovery but also in the restoration of the tissues' morphological and mechanical characteristics after injury. The other key components of rehabilitation include manual therapy, stretching, and neuromuscular exercises. Static stretching[4] and manual joint mobilization[5] each have a strong effect on restoring dorsiflexion after acute ankle sprains. Neuromuscular training, which normally includes balance and coordination exercises, is also supported by the current evidence base. There are consistent data from randomized controlled trials that it can improve functional recovery and prevent reinjury after lateral ankle sprain.[5]

Electrical stimulation can be initiated in the early stages after ankle sprain. It typically involves fixating flexible surface electrodes at or around the injury site with the intention of stimulating the surrounding nerves. Exciting sensory nerves can provide fast symptomatic relief via 2 primary pain-relief mechanisms: the pain-gate mechanism and the endogenous opioid system. By altering the treatment parameters and electrode placements, treatments can also be tailored to electrically stimulate muscle and/or nerves to induce a muscle contraction. This treatment may be particularly useful in the subacute phases after ankle sprain for increasing blood and lymphatic flow, increasing kinesthetic awareness, and improving muscle strength.

Low-level laser therapy (LLLT) is a noninvasive, painless light treatment that is sometimes used in the management of musculoskeletal disorders. The underpinning mechanism is photobioactivation, whereby light, at a single wavelength, is absorbed by the cells at the injury site, producing a wide range of biological events and cellular processes. These processes include modulation of the inflammatory response, fibroblast proliferation, and collagen synthesis. Another popular method for delivering energy to injured tissue is the application of therapeutic ultrasound, which involves the transdermal transmission of mechanical energy in the form of sound waves toward the injured tissue. Ultrasound can have both thermal and athermal effects, with the balance dictated by the treatment parameters. A low-dose pulsed application produces athermal effects that are very similar to those of LLLT, including inflammatory modulation and increased protein synthesis.

The basic premise for using any electrophysical agent after ankle sprain is to transfer energy to the injury site. Theoretically, healing systems should benefit from this energy, but there are numerous parameter combinations available (frequency, intensity, and total dose) and clinically appropriate dosages are often not known. It is also important to note that for any energy-physical intervention to have a positive effect on healing, the energy transmitted to the body must be absorbed efficiently by the tissues. LLLT is preferentially absorbed in superficial vascular tissue, whereas collagen-based tissues such as the lateral ligaments have a higher capacity for absorbing ultrasonic energy. However, the clinical evidence for many electrical agents for the treatment of ankle instability, including LLLT and ultrasound, is generally weak and/or conflicting. Clinicians should also remain cognizant that transferring excessive energy to an injury site can be destructive and therefore deleterious for recovery; as such, a useful guide is to select the lowest intensity that produces a therapeutic response.

Conclusion

Early protection should be replaced with functional management based on early progressive movement for ankle sprains with mild or moderate severity. Cryotherapy has an important adjunctive role during the acute and subacute phases after injury. These roles mainly relate to providing analgesia and facilitating early movement and rehabilitation through cryokinetics. There is conflicting evidence to support the use of other electrophysical agents, which may relate to difficulties in optimal dose selection. NSAIDs should be used with caution after ankle sprain and may be most appropriate when there is significant concomitant synovitits. Simple analgesics such as paracetamol/acetaminophen should be used as an alternative form of pain relief after most ankle sprains. Stretching, manual therapy, and neuromuscular training are effective interventions for normalizing ankle dorsiflexion and minimizing the risk of reinjury. Progressive mechanical loading of the injured tissue offers the best potential to have a specific effect on tissue healing. Future research must continue to develop evidence-based guidelines on a safe, progressive rehabilitation protocol while respecting the time frame associated with ligament healing.

References

1. Kerkhoffs GM, Rowe BH, Assendelft WJ, et al. Immobilisation and functional treatment for acute lateral ankle ligament injuries in adults. *Cochrane Database Syst Rev.* 2002;(3):CD003762.
2. Paoloni JA, Milne C, Orchard J, Hamilton B. Non-steroidal anti-inflammatory drugs in sports medicine: guidelines for practical but sensible use. *Br J Sports Med.* 2009;43:863-865.
3. Bleakley CM, Glasgow PD, Phillips N. Association of Chartered Physiotherapists in Sports and Exercise Medicine (ACPSM). Guidelines on the management of acute soft tissue injury using protection rest ice compression and elevation. London: ACPSM; 2011:15-21.
4. Terada M, Pietrosimone BG, Gribble PA. Therapeutic interventions for increasing ankle dorsiflexion after ankle sprain: a systematic review. *J Athl Train.* 2013;48:696-709.
5. Bleakley CM, McDonough SM, MacAuley DC. Some conservative strategies are effective when added to controlled mobilisation with external support after acute ankle sprain: a systematic review. *Aust J Physiother.* 2008;54:7-20.

HOW MUCH SHOULD I BE CONCERNED ABOUT PERSISTENT LAXITY ASSOCIATED WITH THE LATERAL ANKLE LIGAMENTS?

John E. Kovaleski, PhD, ATC

Lateral ankle laxity commonly results from a tear or lengthening of the anterior talofibular and calcaneofibular ligaments supporting the ankle complex or less-than-optimal healing of the involved tissues. Lateral talocrural (ankle) ligament injury following acute or recurrent lateral ankle sprain can also negatively affect ankle joint motion as evidenced by long-term limitations in dorsiflexion range of motion. During the swing phase of walking, ankle laxity has been shown to disrupt the normal gliding motion and produce anterolateral rotational instability that permits the talus to rotate internally and subluxate anteriorly on the tibia. Furthermore, lateral ankle sprain can damage the ligaments of the talocalcaneal joint and lead to subtalar joint instability.[1]

Ligament Injury and Healing

Partial and complete tears of the lateral ankle ligaments are clinically recognized by the presence of various symptoms that include pain, swelling, edema, difficulty in weight bearing, limited range of motion, and joint instability. Injury occurs when tissue-damaging force exceeds the mechanical strength of the ligament's

McKeon PO, Wikstrom EA, eds. *Quick Questions in Ankle Sprains: Expert Advice in Sports Medicine* (pp 165-169). © 2015 SLACK Incorporated.

fibers. During healing, several biological stages occur that activate the production and movement of cell-producing connective tissue into the injured area. New tissue components form, including immature type III collagen, glycol proteins, and elastin. With ligament healing of a grade III injury (complete tear), a complex series of sequelae occur that form a neoligament, which is more scar-like than the healthy original tissue. The application of mechanical stimuli with mobility exercises spurs the migration of cells that develop and reorient the connective tissue fibers into a layout that helps to strengthen the new tissue. This remodeling process may last months or years, with the injured ligament never fully recovering normal structure and function.[2]

Ligament Laxity Following Lateral Ankle Sprain

Ligament laxity or looseness is measured as joint translation or rotation at a given force or torque and describes the degree of mechanical stability of the ankle complex. Laxity is the most predictable mechanical impairment appearing after lateral ankle sprain and describes a physical or clinical sign that can be objectively detected by manual stress tests, stress radiographs, and instrumented arthrometry. The hypothesis is that laxity leads to instability, and instability leads to disability, which in turn is reflected by an inability to perform functional activities and progressive arthritic changes. Laxity is more easily demonstrated in the chronically unstable ankle, because the joint tends to be less painful.

Altered joint stability characteristics of the ankle complex have been observed in athletes who report a history of lateral ankle sprain.[3] Findings have shown that injured ankles demonstrate mainly increased anterior laxity (Figure 32-1) and greater inversion laxity (Figure 32-2) while displaying reduced anterior and inversion end-range stiffness when measured with an ankle arthrometer. In general, measurement of load and deformation can reflect the structural properties of the ligaments and other soft tissues surrounding the ankle complex. When performing a physical examination following a sprain, end-range stiffness or end-feel identifies the nature of resistance that is felt at the limits of the joint's end range of motion. End-feel acts as a measure of the elasticity of tissue that can be quantified as the mechanical property of stiffness, which in turn provides a measure of the end range of the supporting tissue's elasticity that includes the secondary soft-tissue structures and any affected capsuloligamentous structures surrounding the joint. Because soft tissue is more compliant at low loads, higher force loads increase the tissues' stiffness as unit increases in force are produced. The lack of a solid endpoint indicates

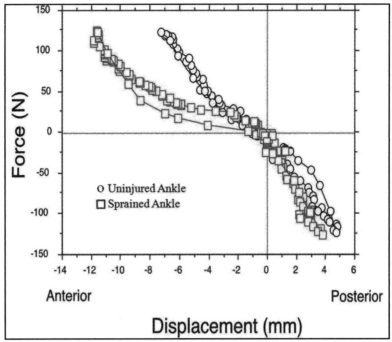

Figure 32-1. Bilateral anteroposterior force-displacement curves showing an uninjured and a laterally sprained (lax) ankle. Observe the increased anterior laxity (mm) of the sprained versus the uninjured ankle.

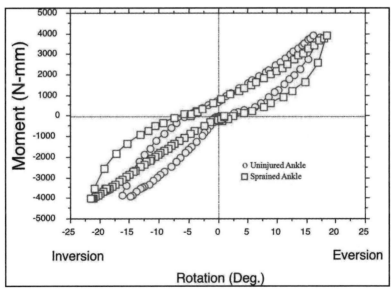

Figure 32-2. Bilateral inversion-eversion load-displacement curves showing an uninjured and a laterally sprained (lax) ankle. Observe the increased inversion laxity (range of motion [degrees]) of the sprained (lax) versus the uninjured ankle.

that the ligamentous structures are injured and any resulting end-feel is likely produced by the intact structures that support the joint.[4]

When ligaments do not heal appropriately and laxity persists, alterations in the passive tension (elasticity) characteristics of the soft tissues surrounding the ankle complex occur and lead to the development of ankle pathologies. These changes to the biophysical properties of the ligament and secondary support tissues of the ankle complex could explain the increased laxity and altered end-feel characteristics observed in individuals who report a history of ankle sprain. Clinically, this can lead to joint instability due to the progressive stretching of the healing ligament scar during early activity or rehabilitation. The biomechanical explanation for this "stretching out" is "irrecoverable creep," which has been demonstrated as deformation or elongation under a constant load that is not recovered following unloading of the ligament.[5]

If return to activity is permitted before the ligament is fully healed, the ligament may heal in a lax or elongated state. These effects on the ligament appear to be biologic in nature and involve changes in extracellular matrix composition, decreased collagen fibril diameter size, and reduced collagen cross links. This elongated ligament state could result in tissue-stiffness changes that over time lead to the involvement of sensorimotor impairments. Athletes with mechanical instability may not always present with clinical symptoms because their neuromotor capabilities are able to provide the necessary supportive restraint, especially in the presence of near-normal ankle range of motion and end-feel. Functional instability is linked to impaired proprioception, altered neuromuscular control, ankle-strength deficits, and diminished postural control. By contrast, pain resulting from other pathology caused by anatomic changes can produce symptoms similar to those of functional ankle instability in the patient without laxity. One must maintain a high level of suspicion for other associated injuries when evaluating these patients, as this will affect treatment recommendations.

Developing a better understanding of the effects of acute and recurrent ankle sprains on ligament laxity is important, because poorly managed ankle ligament injuries can lead to mechanical instability and long-term complications. Described as a clinical symptom, mechanical ankle instability is associated with a lax or unstable ankle following ligament injury that is measured as motion beyond the normal physiological or accessory range of joint motion. Mechanical instability results from specific insufficiencies such as laxity caused by a sprain, arthrokinematic restriction, synovial irritation, and degenerative changes within the joints of the ankle complex.[1,3] Other, unknown sequelae that induce changes to other structures if there is failure to protect the ligament could also develop.[2,5] The dilemma for the clinician is to find what is causing the dysfunction by watching for abnormal joint movement, increased range of motion, joint swelling for no apparent reason, giving way of the ankle, or the presence of an abnormal end-feel.

Conclusion

Immediate care and rehabilitation should focus on enhancing ligament healing following ankle sprain. During rehabilitation, the optimal loading environment for a ligament scar may be critical to its long-term strength. Early protection through immobilization and brace support to therapeutic exercise helps the newly laid-down collagen align with the forces of the ankle. Persistent ligamentous laxity may be due to inappropriate care and rehabilitation, which compels the need for new study into the types of care and treatment that will best promote tissue healing while enhancing joint stability and maximizing normal joint function. Our present understanding based on available evidence supports the concern that persistent laxity associated with the lateral ligaments is a clinical problem that is associated with a variety of ankle complex impairments, such as mechanical and chronic ankle instability.

References

1. Kovaleski, JE, Hollis JM, Heitman RJ, Gurchiek LR, Pearsall AW. Assessment of ankle-subtalar joint complex laxity using an instrumented ankle arthrometer: an experimental cadaveric investigation. *J Athl Train*. 2002;37:467-474.
2. Chamberlain CS, Crowley EM, Kobayashi H, Eliceiri KW, Vanderby R. Quantification of collagen organization and extracellular matrix factors within the healing ligament. *Microsc Microanal*. 2011;17:779-787.
3. Cordova ML, Sefton JM, Hubbard TJ. Mechanical joint laxity associated with chronic ankle instability: a systematic review. *Sports Health*. 2010;2:452-459.
4. Kovaleski JE, Heitman RJ, Gurchiek LR, et al. Joint stability characteristics of the ankle complex in female athletes with histories of lateral ankle sprain, part II: clinical experience using arthrometric measurement. *J Athl Train*. 2014;49:198-203.
5. Majima T, Lo IKY, Marchuk LL, Shrive NG, Frank CB. Effects of ligament repair on laxity and creep behavior of an early healing ligament scar. *J Orthop Sci*. 2006;11:272-277.

WHAT SHOULD BE CONSIDERED WHEN REHABILITATING A PEDIATRIC ANKLE SPRAIN?

Claire E. Hiller, PhD, MAppSc, BAppSc (Physio) and
Joshua Burns, PhD, BAppSc (Pod)(Hons)

It is often tempting to dismiss a pediatric sprain as a simple injury that will have no long-lasting effect and therefore require no treatment. However, a recent systematic review of chronic ankle instability, which is a common residual problem from an ankle sprain, illustrated the high prevalence of instability and recurrent sprain in children.[1] Many of these children had an ankle sprain in their early years, and the residual problems had lasted for more than 12 years. Surveys of adults also highlight that many long-term problems began with an ankle sprain in childhood.[2] So, careful rehabilitation should be implemented no matter at what age the sprain occurs.

The rehabilitation of a pediatric ankle sprain is essentially the same as that for an adult. The main differences to consider are the child's age and developmental stage, equipment (Figure 33-1) and outcome measures, and the unresolved sprain. Rehabilitation of ankle sprains in children requires consideration and knowledge of the stages of cognitive, physical, and motor control development. In the younger child, many clues will have been gained from the assessment to assist with planning and modifying the rehabilitation program. The level of language and communication observed will guide the clinician in assessing the ability of the child to articulate pain or discomfort with exercises or the ability to comprehend what is

McKeon PO, Wikstrom EA, eds. *Quick Questions in
Ankle Sprains: Expert Advice in Sports Medicine* (pp 171-174).
© 2015 SLACK Incorporated.

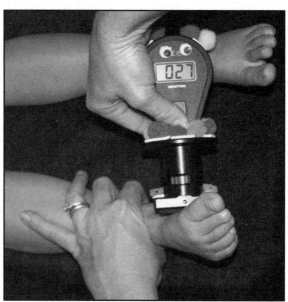

Figure 33-1. Modified dynamometer for use with young children.

expected. Other important clues are the poise and confidence of the child, which indicate the likelihood of being compliant with treatment, the child's attention span, and distractibility.[3] The level and style of parental involvement during the assessment will aid the clinician in discerning the level of support likely for a rehabilitation program. It is useful for patients at any age to have clearly established goals for rehabilitation, discussed in conjunction with the parent/caregiver, child, and clinician. Joint negotiation will open the discussion regarding aims, prognosis, progressions, and awareness of potential red flags.[3]

Rehabilitation should be planned according to the child's individual development and motor control rather than his or her age. Although age will give some guidance about physiological capacity, there can be a wide variation in physical maturation in children of the same age.[4] However, all aspects of rehabilitation can be implemented, even in the very young.

Restoration of muscle strength around the ankle can be implemented in patients as young as 5 years.[4] Before puberty, strength is primarily directed by neural adaptation, while adolescents increase strength through increasing cross-sectional area with neural adaptations, similar to adults.[4] Therefore, ankle-strength work that aims to increase ankle muscle mass is inappropriate in the preadolescent.

Balance retraining is often used in ankle sprain rehabilitation. The ability to balance is a motor skill that develops throughout childhood, and an extended single-leg balance with the eyes closed, a mainstay of ankle rehabilitation, is often not possible before the age of 9 years. Balance control appears to shift from large-amplitude ballistic adjustments to smoother quicker adjustments with age. Children show less anteroposterior stability, possibly due to an underdeveloped ankle strategy.[5] At around 10 years of age, simple balance strategies are similar to those of adults; however, when more challenging tasks are attempted, strategies revert to those of an earlier developmental stage.[5] Thus, the clinician should not expect to retrain an efficient ankle strategy with small smooth oscillation control when rehabilitating children. In addition, the clinician can expect an apparent regression when progressing balance tasks which may be due to an underdeveloped ankle strategy and not solely due to the extra challenge.

Restoration of functional activity should be in line with motor development, so the clinician working with young children needs to be aware of the major developmental milestones and to structure rehabilitation aims accordingly. Creativity and flexibility are the hallmarks for functional rehabilitation, as it is the rare child who can happily concentrate for the time required to perform routine rehabilitation tasks. Engagement in rehabilitation using fun functional tasks or Wii Fit training-type electronic activities will serve the clinician better than repetitive Thera-Band or balance activities.

Some consideration should be given to the adolescent who is undergoing a growth spurt. It appears that while motor skills may not be affected during this time, specific aspects of motor control (ie, postural stability, neuromuscular control, and intersegmental coordination) might be affected.[4] There may also be a regression in the adolescent's ability to integrate proprioceptive inputs, and so there is an increased reliance on visual cues.[4] While these effects are highly individual, the clinician should be aware that rehabilitation may not progress as quickly as expected during this time.

Pediatric-specific outcome measures should be employed when possible. While adolescents are similar to adults with many measures, younger children will require developmentally appropriate goals in functional and balance measures. There is currently only one pediatric outcome measure for chronic ankle instability.[1] The Cumberland ankle instability tool—youth (CAITY), which is an adaptation of the CAIT, has been developed and validated for children aged from 8 years and older. The CAITY measures the child's perception of how unstable his or her ankle feels on a scale of 0 to 30, with 0 indicating severe instability and 30 indicating no instability.

Mention should be made that children usually recover quickly from an ankle sprain, although a quick recovery does not preclude long-term ankle problems. If a complaint is made of ongoing pain, or an increase or return of pain following a period of improvement, the clinician should be suspicious of a comorbidity, which may include an osteochondral injury or tarsal coalition[3] (refer to Question 19).

References

1. Mandarakas M, Pourkazemi F, Sman A, Burns J, Hiller CE. Systematic review of chronic ankle instability in children. *J Foot Ankle Res.* 2014:7:21.
2. Hiller CE, Nightingale EJ, Raymond J, et al. Prevalence and impact of chronic musculoskeletal ankle disorders in the community. *Arch Phys Med Rehabil.* 2012:93:1801-1807.
3. Burns J, Redmond AC, Hunt J. Childhood disorders of the foot and lower limb. New York: Nova Science Publishers, Inc; 2012.
4. Lloyd RS, Faigenbaum AD, Stone MH, et al. Position statement on youth resistance training: the 2014 international consensus. *Br J Sports Med.* 2014;48:498-505.
5. Quatman-Yates CC, Quatman CE, Meszaros AJ, Paterno MV, Hewett TE. A systematic review of sensorimotor function during adolescence: a developmental stage of increased motor awkwardness? *Br J Sports Med.* 2012:46:649-655.

WHAT ARE THE MOST APPROPRIATE PATIENT-ORIENTED OUTCOME MEASURES TO USE FOR GAUGING DISABILITY AND FUNCTIONAL RECOVERY DURING REHABILITATION FOLLOWING ANKLE SPRAIN?

Todd A. Evans, PhD, ATC and Kelli R. Snyder, EdD, ATC

Following an ankle sprain, patients typically experience some loss of ability and function. As clinicians, our goal through rehabilitation is to help these patients restore their ability and to regain function. Whereas measuring impairments such as tissue healing, range of motion, and joint laxity during recovery provide us with physiological reference points, they do not represent patient ability or function. Therefore, to the patient, they can be meaningless. Outcomes that are meaningful to the patient are referred to as patient-oriented (patient-centered) outcomes and reflect the patient's interests and recovery goals. They address the patient's quality of life and reflect what they want to do, what they are able to do, their symptoms, and how they are able to function in their environment. Examples include pain and the ability to work, exercise, take part in recreational activities, and perform activities of daily living (ADL). By identifying and monitoring patient-oriented outcomes during recovery from ankle sprains, we can optimize individual patient

McKeon PO, Wikstrom EA, eds. *Quick Questions in Ankle Sprains: Expert Advice in Sports Medicine* (pp 175-178).
© 2015 SLACK Incorporated.

care and ultimately improve the effectiveness of our interventions. Identifying which patient-oriented outcomes to measure, however, is much less challenging than determining how to measure them. The purpose of this chapter is to identify the most appropriate patient-oriented outcome measures to use for gauging disability and functional recovery during rehabilitation following ankle sprain.

Appropriate patient-oriented measures address the important clinical constructs from the patient's perspective. The universally accepted format for assessing patient-oriented outcomes is through patient-reported outcome (PRO) measures. These instruments are designed to quantify a patient's health status by having the patient respond to a list of questions (items). Items address specific symptoms or components of ability and function, and provide the patient with Likert-type response choices representing a range of intensities (eg, from severe problem to no problem; from no difficulty to unable to perform). Each response option is assigned a point value, and the sum of the responses produces a total score. Because there is no PRO specific to recovery following ankle sprains, using a region-specific PRO is the best option. There are, however, more than 50 region-specific outcome measures available for the ankle and foot. Although each measure was created to quantify a patient's health status following ankle/foot pathology, each is different in its construction, administration, validation, and application. To provide clarity, Martin and Irrgang[1] identified 5 region-specific ankle/foot PRO instruments with adequate evidence supporting the standard measurement properties of validity, reliability, and responsiveness.[1,2] They included the foot and ankle ability measure (FAAM), foot function index (FFI), foot health status questionnaire (FHSQ), lower-extremity functional scale (LEFS), and the sports ankle rating system quality-of-life measure (SARS-QOL).

Of the 5 region-specific PRO instruments that Martin and Irrgang[1] identified, the best option for gauging ability and function during recovery from an ankle sprain appears to be the FAAM. Although not specifically designed for ankle sprains, the FAAM has evidence of validity for general ankle, foot, and lower-leg musculoskeletal pathologies, including sprains.[3] It consists of 2 subscales that are scored separately: (1) a 21-item activities of daily living subscale, and (2) an 8-item sports subscale. The FAAM is a revised version of the foot and ankle disability index (FADI) and has evidence to support its content and construct validity, as well as its reliability and responsiveness.[3] The FAAM offers Likert-type responses ranging from a score of 4 (no difficulty) to 0 (unable to do), in addition to an NA (not applicable) response option. Final subscale scores are calculated as percentages of a patient's total possible score with NA responses excluded. For example, if a patient's ADL subscale response total is 40, but the responses included 2 NA responses, then the maximum ADL score is 76 (4 × 19 instead of 4 × 21), with a final calculated ADL subscale score as 53% (40 of 76). The minimal clinically important difference for the scales is 8% for the ADL and 9% for the sport subscale.[3]

One of the unique features of the FAAM is the inclusion of a sports subscale. These questions offer the potential to minimize a ceiling effect because the items represent higher levels of ability and function. Ceiling effects are a common issue with these types of instruments and occur when the items do not match the ability and function of the patient. Patients therefore can achieve a maximum score before they have returned to preinjury ability and functional levels. The consequence is that the patient may truly continue to have deficits in function and ability, but his or her score already represents the maximum score. Any improvement in function or ability would therefore not be represented by the instrument because the patient cannot score any higher. Although the FAAM has adequate validity for a general population of patients, it has not been specifically validated for patients with higher levels of ability, such as elite athletes and other patients with extremely high levels of physical ability.

A solution to address potential ceiling effects with region-specific PROs is incorporating a patient-specific functional scale (PSFS).[4,5] Unlike a region-specific instrument, which consists of a predetermined set of questions, a PSFS is created by the patient during the initial rehabilitation session. To create a PSFS, the patient is guided by the clinician to identify at least 3 (no more than 5) meaningful activities that are currently limited because of his or her ankle sprain. The patient is then asked to rate his or her current difficulty for each activity on an 11-point scale, usually from 0 (unable to perform) to 10 (able to perform before injury), and these responses are recorded by the clinician for that date. Then, during subsequent sessions, the clinician guides the patient through listed activities and records scores for each, from 0 to 10. In addition to the initial items being specific to each patient, there is the option of adding additional activities (items) that are limited but were not identified in the initial session. These additional items typically represent more difficult activities that were not apparent or considered by the patient in the initial stage of recovery. The obvious advantage for the PSFS is its specificity to the individual patient. The PSFS has evidence of validity for both the clinical setting and in outcomes research.[4,5] A disadvantage of a PSFS is that it is not intended to be a comprehensive PRO and does not typically incorporate items representing pain and other basic activities that are important to address but may not have been identified by the patient. It is therefore meant to complement a region-specific instrument such as the FAAM, and the combination of the 2 instruments may offer the ideal patient-oriented outcome measure for gauging recovery following an ankle sprain.

Whereas systematic monitoring of outcomes can help shape and improve recovery following ankle sprain, the most important reason/justification for assessing and monitoring PROs is the health and welfare of the individual patient. The use of PROs is efficient, important, useful, and accepted throughout health care. Using the FAAM combined with a PSFS offers the most appropriate patient-oriented ankle sprain outcome measure for gauging disability and functional recovery during rehabilitation.

References

1. Martin RL, Irrgang JJ. A survey of self-reported outcome instruments for the foot and ankle. *J Orthop Sports Phys Ther.* 2007;37:72-84.
2. Reeve BB, Wyrwich KW, Wu AW, et. al. ISOQOL recommends minimum standards for patient-reported outcome measures used in patient-centered outcomes and comparative effectiveness research. *Qual Life Res.* 2013;22:1889-1905.
3. Martin RL, Irrgang JJ, Burdett RG, Conti SF, Van Swearingen JM. Evidence of validity for the foot and ankle ability measure (FAAM). *Foot Ankle Int.* 2005;26:968-983.
4. Horn KK, Jennings S, Richardson G, Vliet DV, Hefford C, Abbott JH. The patient-specific functional scale: psychometrics, clinimetrics, and application as a clinical outcome measure. *J Orthop Sports Phys Ther.* 2012;42:30-42.
5. Abbott JH, Schmitt JS. The patient-specific functional scale was valid for group-level change comparisons and between-group discrimination. *J Clin Epidemiol.* 2014;pii:S0895-4356(13)00472-1. doi: 10.1016/j.jclinepi.2013.11.002.

SECTION IV

SURGICAL CONSIDERATIONS

WHEN SHOULD I REFER MY PATIENT WITH AN ANKLE PROBLEM TO AN ORTHOPEDIC SURGEON?

Kelli Frye Pugh, MS, ATC, LMT

Ankle injuries are a common orthopedic injury seen by health care providers. Athletic trainers, family practice physicians, or emergency department physicians are frequently the first health care provider to evaluate such injuries. Not all patients with ankle injuries need referral, but health care providers should perform a systematic, thorough evaluation. Certain objective findings require timely referral, as do some at-risk patient populations.

The initial evaluation of an ankle injury includes taking a history, followed by observation and palpation. The patient's history can provide an indication of the mechanism of injury and potentially the structures injured. Unfortunately, not all patients will be able to provide an accurate history of the mechanism of injury. Clinicians should next turn to observation of the foot, ankle, and lower leg, looking for deformity, edema, effusion, and ecchymosis. Any gross deformity should be immediately splinted, and the patient should be referred to an orthopedist. However, it is important to consider that not all patients with ankle fractures present with gross deformity. Many patients with ankle injury present with edema or effusion, but swelling alone is not an indicator of injury severity.[1] Ankle edema is less concerning than a true joint effusion, which could indicate a chondral lesion or syndesmotic injury and would warrant referral. Patients with syndesmotic injuries typically present with pain at the anterior inferior tibiofibular ligament that extends

McKeon PO, Wikstrom EA, eds. *Quick Questions in*
Ankle Sprains: Expert Advice in Sports Medicine (pp 181-184).
© 2015 SLACK Incorporated.

superiorly into the syndesmosis. Chondral injuries can involve a more diffuse pain in the talocrural joint that is difficult for the patient to localize with palpation.

Palpation should include the lower leg, ankle, and foot. The Ottawa ankle rules (OAR)[2] provide a highly sensitive, well-validated, and clinically useful tool for determining the necessity of radiographs for the foot and ankle following acute injury. The OAR state that an ankle radiograph is needed if the patient reports pain near the malleoli and one or more of the following criteria are met: age 55 years or older, unable to bear weight both immediately after the injury and at time of examination (4 steps, regardless of pain or limping), or bone tenderness of the tibia or fibula along the distal 6 cm of the posterior edge or at the inferior tip of the malleolus. A radiograpgh of the foot is needed if the patient reports pain in the midfoot area and there is bony tenderness at the navicular, cuboid, or base of the fifth metatarsal. Ankle injuries can sometimes involve concomitant foot injuries, such as a Jones fracture, Lisfranc sprain, midfoot sprain, or bone bruise to the adjacent tarsal bones, which require further evaluation.

Leddy et al[3] proposed a modification to the OAR, called the Buffalo rule, which moves the area of palpation to the crests of the distal 6 cm of the tibia and fibula (instead of the posterior edge). The other criteria of the original OAR remain the same. This modification was made to minimize palpating the ligamentous attachments at the posterior edges of the malleoli (Table 35-1). Patients who meet the criteria of the OAR, or the Buffalo rule modification, should be referred to an orthopedic surgeon for further evaluation. The patient should also be referred if the clinician's ability to accurately palpate bony structures is compromised as a result of accumulated edema.

Any patient with an acute ankle injury that is not improving with rest and treatment after several days should be referred to an orthopedist for evaluation. Certain populations and pathologies also require special consideration for referral. Geriatric or osteoporotic patients have increased fracture risk. Pediatric patients with immature bone are at risk for epiphyseal injuries, or Salter-Harris fractures. Syndesmotic ankle sprains, or "high ankle sprains," also require special consideration and a more conservative management approach than that for lateral ankle sprains. While none is well validated, special ligamentous tests for syndesmotic sprain include the squeeze test, Cotton test, external-rotation test (Kleiger's test), and fibular translation test.[4,5] It is important for the orthopedist to evaluate the integrity of the ankle mortise with plain radiographs and/or magnetic resonance imaging following a suspected syndesmotic injury.

Recurrent ankle injury or chronic ankle instability provide unique management challenges. While edema is difficult to completely resolve following acute ankle injury, any patient with fluctuant ankle swelling and lingering pain should raise concern for a clinician. Examples of ankle pathologies that may cause chronic

Table 35-1 OAR²/Buffalo Rule Modification³	
An ankle radiograph is needed if there is pain near the malleoli AND one or more of the following are seen:	**A foot radiograph is needed if there is pain in the midfoot AND:**
• Age 55 years or older • Unable to bear weight, both immediately and at evaluation; 4 steps, regardless of limp • Bone tenderness along the distal 6 cm of the posterior edge of the tibia or at the inferior tip of the medial malleolus (Buffalo modification; tenderness along the distal 6 cm of the crest of the tibia and inferior tip of the malleolus) • Bone tenderness along the distal 6 cm of the posterior edge of the fibula or at the inferior tip of the lateral malleolus (Buffalo modification; tenderness along the distal 6 cm of the crest of the fibula and inferior tip of the malleolus)	• Bone tenderness at the navicular, cuboid, or base of the fifth metatarsal
Exclusion criteria in the OAR included chronic injury (more than 10 days old), pregnancy, presence of isolated injuries to the skin (lacerations, abrasions, etc), and under 18 years of age.	

problems include arthritis, chondral lesions, functional ligamentous instability, os trigonum syndrome, and soft-tissue injuries to the peroneal or Achilles tendon.[5] Physician management for these conditions can include advanced diagnostic imaging and, potentially, surgical intervention. A patient who has failed 3 to 6 months of conservative treatment, whose injury causes pain during activities of daily living, or who has complaints of recurrent instability or swelling, should be referred to an orthopedist for consideration of an ankle ligament repair or reconstruction. In the athletic population, these patients may remain highly functional but complain of pain, a subjective lack of power, and feelings of instability during running and cutting activities.

Finally, the patient's anxiety over the injury should be taken into account. While most sports medicine clinicians are very familiar with ankle injuries and the expected course of recovery, it may be the patient's first experience with such an injury. A referral to an orthopedist is sometimes warranted to provide reassurance that there is no fracture and that the symptoms the person is experiencing are typical.

A number of factors require consideration to determine when a clinician should refer a patient with an ankle problem to an orthopedic surgeon. While any patient with obvious deformity should be referred for further evaluation, the amount of swelling is not necessarily an accurate indicator of injury severity. The OAR, with the addition of the Buffalo rule modification, provides a highly sensitive, objective basis for the necessity of radiologic examination and should be used in the clinical decision-making process. Elderly and pediatric patients require special consideration for referral given their unique fracture risk as a result of either osteoporotic or immature bone. Syndesmotic ankle sprains offer a different set of management concerns. Patients with chronic instability or increasing ankle dysfunction warrant physician referral for an evaluation of additional pathology. A patient whose injury has failed 3 to 6 months of conservative management and has ongoing complaints of pain, swelling, or instability should be referred for potential surgical ligament repair/reconstruction. Also, the patient's affect and level of anxiety regarding the injury should be considered.

References

1. Sujitkumar P, Hadfield JM, Yates DW. Sprain or fracture: an analysis of 2000 ankle injuries. *Arch Emerg Med.* 1986;3:101-106.
2. Stiell IG, Greenberg GH, Mcknight RD, et al. A study to develop clinical decision rules for the use of radiography in acute ankle injuries. *Ann Emerg Med.* 1992;21:384-390.
3. Leddy JJ, Smolinski RJ, Lawrence J, Snyder JL, Priore RL. Prospective evaluation of the Ottawa ankle rules in a university sports medicine center: with a modification to increase specificity for identifying malleolar fractures. *Am J Sport Med.* 1998;26:158-165.
4. Kaminski TW, Hertel J, Amendola N, et al. National Athletic Trainers' Association position statement: conservative management and prevention of ankle sprains in athletes. *J Athl Train.* 2013;48:528-545.
5. Starkey C, Brown SD, Ryan JL. *Examination of Orthopedic and Athletic Injuries.* 3rd ed. Philadelphia, PA: F.A. Davis; 2010:249-265.

WHICH SURGICAL TECHNIQUE PRODUCES THE BEST CLINICAL OUTCOMES IN LATERAL ANKLE SPRAINS?

Chad M. Ferguson, MD and J. Kent Ellington, MD, MS

Lateral ankle sprains are among the most common injuries incurred during sports participation. Conservative management of lateral ankle sprains with traditional methods is the mainstay of treatment for acute and chronic lateral ankle sprains. After evaluation of a patient with persistent symptoms following failed conservative management of lateral ankle sprain, there is a host of procedures that have been suggested for surgical treatment.

Patient Evaluation and Surgical Indications

Surgical decision making depends on persistent complaints of subjective instability, demonstrable positive physical examination findings, and radiographic signs correlating with ankle instability. Patients typically present with subjective complaints of instability of the ankle with recurrent lateral ankle sprains occurring with running and cutting activities or with walking on uneven surfaces and are persistent despite efforts toward activity modification or bracing.

Positive physical examination findings need also to be present to indicate surgery. The anterior drawer test is conducted by the examiner holding the tibia above

McKeon PO, Wikstrom EA, eds. *Quick Questions in Ankle Sprains: Expert Advice in Sports Medicine* (pp 185-190).

the level of the ankle in a stationary position while imparting an anterior directed force on the talus and calcaneus. The inversion stress test is conducted by placing an inward stress on the talus while holding the tibia stationary. A positive result from either of these tests is a finding of increased laxity compared to that on the contralateral side. Additionally, while performing these provocative tests, a slight depression may form over the lateral aspect of the ankle, known as the sulcus sign.

Radiographs, including anteroposterior, lateral, and mortise weight-bearing views, should also be obtained. In patients with positive physical examination findings, stress inversion radiographs showing more than 15 degrees of talar tilt and stress anterior drawer radiographs showing greater than 1 cm anterior translation confirm the diagnosis of ankle instability.

For patients meeting these diagnostic criteria, conservative treatment with a functional rehabilitation physical therapy protocol complete with range of motion, proprioception, strengthening, and bracing should be initiated. With this conservative management, 85% of patients experience resolution of their instability symptoms and do not require long-term external bracing for return to athletic competition; however, 15% of patients develop recurrent instability despite nonsurgical treatment. These patients have recurrent instability episodes and may also have concomitant injuries such as synovitis, impingement, osteochondral defects, deltoid ligament attenuation, peroneal tendon pathology, or loose body formation that contribute to their recalcitrant symptoms.[1] These patients meet the surgical indication, as they have met the diagnostic criteria and failed conservative management.

Procedures

All procedures strive for restoration of the stability of the lateral ankle ligamentous complex. Lateral ankle ligamentous stability primarily depends on 3 principal ligaments: the anterior talofibular ligament (ATFL), the calcaneofibular ligament (CFL), and the posterior talofibular ligament (PTFL). The ATFL and PTFL are discrete structures within the ankle joint capsule, while the CFL is a confluence of the floor of the peroneal tendon sheath. ATFL strain increases as the foot moves into plantar flexion and inversion, while the CFL is strained with increasing degrees of dorsiflexion and inversion due to their anatomic sites of insertion. The inferior extensor retinaculum serves to prevent bowstringing of the long extensor tendons to the foot distal to the ankle. Due to ligamentous biomechanical properties and orientation with respect to the ankle, the ATFL is the most commonly injured, followed by combined injuries of the ATFL and CFL. The PTFL most commonly remains intact after lateral ligamentous injuries.

Cumulative outcomes of lateral ankle surgeries include greater than 80% clinical success.[1] Procedures for treating lateral ankle instability are subcategorized as anatomic or nonanatomic reconstructions. Biomechanical data support anatomic reconstruction to restore ligamentous forces to normal over nonanatomic procedures that seek to restore ankle stability with tendon augmentation procedures.[2]

Anatomic repairs strive to reconstruct the normal anatomy by imbricating the existing joint capsule and attenuated lateral ligaments. The most commonly advocated anatomic surgical procedure for chronic lateral ankle instability from ankle sprain is the Bröstrom-Gould procedure. This procedure addresses the lateral ligamentous laxity caused by chronic lateral ankle sprains by direct reconstruction and augmentation of the native lateral ligaments (hence "anatomic repair"). In this procedure, a lateral incision is made over the ATFL and CFL. Dissection is conducted to first isolate the inferior extensor retinaculum at the level of the distal fibula. This layer is protected for later incorporation. Subsequently, deeper exploration reveals the remaining portion of the damaged and elongated ATFL and the CFL, which are dissected. If the CFL is found to be intact, the surgeon may elect to address only the ATFL. Classically, the Bröstrom procedure uses a pants-over-vest imbrication of attenuated ligaments using nonabsorbable sutures. This repair technique involves overlapping the stretched tissue to facilitate tightening of the structure. The development of suture anchors and other technical modifications such as bone tunnels have allowed surgeons other alternatives to this classic repair. Regardless of the fixation technique, the ATFL sutures are tightened with the patient's foot in eversion and dorsiflexion and with the ankle posteriorly translated to ensure that ligament tension is adequately restored. An important modification to the original Bröstrom procedure is the Gould modification, in which the inferior extensor retinaculum is oversewn superficial to the ligamentous repair to augment the lateral ankle tissues. The wound is closed, and the patient is immobilized for 4 to 6 weeks and progressed to full activity after 12 weeks (Figure 36-1).[3]

Outcomes of the Bröstrom-Gould anatomic lateral ankle reconstruction have shown 85% to 95% good-to-excellent results.[4] This procedure touts stability by reinforcing local host anatomy and maintenance of physiologic lateral tissue motion. Additionally, there is minimal morbidity, as patients do not require harvesting of a local autograft tendon or risk of allograft utilization. Patient-directed outcome variables such as range of motion, strength, complications, reoperation, and return to sport have all been evaluated and found to be excellent. Patients with unsatisfactory results following this procedure have tended to have long-standing ligamentous insufficiency, generalized ligamentous laxity, significant peroneal dysfunction, intra-articular pathology, or deformity.

A novel technique to modify the Bröstrom-Gould repair augments the anatomic repair with nonbiologic tissue. This technique uses a fiber tape construct to overlay

Figure 36-1. (A) Anatomy of the superficial peroneal nerve branches in relationship to the Bröstrom anatomic repair incision (dotted lines). (B) Midsubstance tear of the ATFL and CFL. (C) The Bröstrom ligament repair of the ATFL and CFL. (D) The Gould modification of the Bröstrom ligament repair, mobilizing the proximal aspect of the inferior extensor retinaculum. (Reprinted with permission from Baumhauer JF, O'Brien T. Surgical considerations in the treatment of ankle instability. *J Athl Train*. 2002;37:458-462.)

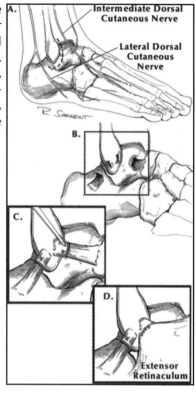

the ATFL. This procedure is added after completion of the Bröstrom repair. A drill hole is placed in the fibula and talus at the respective attachments of the ATFL. Fiber tape is secured with the ankle in slight plantar flexion and inversion to prevent overtightening. Although in its infancy, we speculate that this technique may expedite rehabilitation and serve to back up a tissue repair with a permanent checkrein to prevent recurrence (Figure 36-2).

Nonanatomic procedures using tendons or other grafts for lateral ankle stabilization have been proposed. The Evans procedure is performed by using the anterior 25% to 50% of the peroneus brevis tendon transferred through a bone tunnel to the distal fibula. This procedure maintains the posterior portion of the tendon in its anatomic position to allow continued function of the peroneus brevis muscle. The transferred anterior band effectively forms a checkrein between the peroneus brevis native insertion of the fifth metatarsal base and the lateral distal fibula. This procedure is rarely used in isolation due to poor long-term results, but it has been as a supplementation to the Bröstrom-Gould reconstruction, as it prevents reconstruction failure from subsequent injury in high-risk patients. Care must be taken with this augmentation technique to avoid overtightening with the peroneus brevis transfer (Figure 36-3).

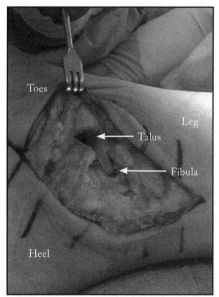

Figure 36-2. Photograph of internal brace placement to augment the anatomic reconstruction with insertion into the distal fibula and talar neck. The white arrows indicate the fiber tape internal brace. (Reprinted with permission of Dr. J. Kent Ellington.)

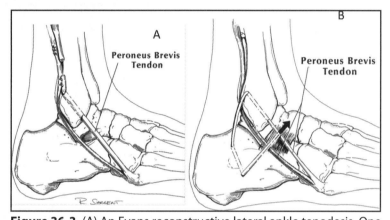

Figure 36-3. (A) An Evans reconstructive lateral ankle tenodesis. One half of the proximal peroneus brevis tendon is harvested, leaving it attached distally to the fifth metatarsal base. The proximal end is weaved anterior to posterior through a drill hole in the fibula and sutured to itself. (B) The Chrisman-Snook reconstructive lateral ankle tenodesis. One half of the proximal aspect of the peroneus brevis tendon is harvested, leaving it attached distally to the fifth metatarsal base. The proximal tendon is weaved anterior to posterior through a drill hole in the fibula and posterior to anterior in a calcaneal bone tunnel and sutured to itself in the region of the anterior talofibular ligament. (Reprinted with permission from Baumhauer JF, O'Brien T. Surgical considerations in the treatment of ankle instability. *J Athl Train*. 2002;37:458-462.)

Another nonanatomic reconstruction has been proposed using the peroneus brevis muscle. Known as the Chrisman-Snook procedure, this procedure detaches the anterior 50% of the peroneus brevis tendon at its myotendinous junction proximally. The distal insertion maintains its attachment to the base of the fifth metatarsal, like in the Evans procedure. The tendon is then weaved from anterior to posterior obliquely through the distal fibula and then through the lateral calcaneus and finally is inserted on the lateral talar neck at the native insertion of the ATFL. A major critique of the original procedure is that it results in restriction of subtalar motion and subjective "tightness" perceived by patients. When this procedure was compared to the Bröstrom-Gould procedure, significantly increased complications, including sural nerve injuries, restriction of physiologic motion, and wound problems were found in the patient group who underwent the Chrisman-Snook procedure.[1] Contraindications for anatomic lateral ligament reconstructions include patients with neurologic or neuromuscular disorders, those who have failed a primary reconstruction, or those who require a salvage lateral ankle stabilization. Additionally, special considerations exist for patients who weigh more than 250 pounds and those with hindfoot varus, constitutional ligamentous laxity, or concomitant peroneal tendon disorders. For these patients, nonanatomic procedures as well as other reconstructive options provide viable solutions to correct chronic instability during the primary surgery.[1,4]

Conclusion

Chronic lateral ankle instability due to ankle sprain is a condition that is successfully managed conservatively in the majority of cases. When patients fail conservative measures, surgical intervention with anatomic ligament reconstruction with the Bröstrom-Gould procedure is the preferred technique for providing durable and functional results, restoring the patient's ankle stability, and providing pain relief. Additional techniques are available and are used in primary and revision settings at the surgeon's discretion.

References

1. Clanton TO, McGarvey W. Chapter 26: Athletic injuries to the soft tissues of the foot and ankle. In: Coughlin MJ, Mann RA, Saltzman CL. *Surgery of the Foot and Ankle*. Philadelphia, PA: Mosby; 2007.
2. Bahr R, Pena F, Shine J, et al: Biomechanics of ankle ligament reconstruction: an in vitro comparison of the Bröstrom repair, Watson-Jones reconstruction, and a new anatomic reconstruction technique. *Am J Sports Med*. 1997;25:424-432.
3. Wiesel SW. *Operative Techniques in Orthopaedic Surgery*. Philadelphia, PA: Lippincott Williams & Wilkins; 2010.
4. Baumhauer JF, O'Brien T. Surgical considerations in the treatment of ankle instability. *J Athl Train*. 2002;37:458-462.

WHAT ARE THE KEY REHABILITATION CONSIDERATIONS FOR PRODUCING THE BEST CLINICAL OUTCOMES FOLLOWING LATERAL ANKLE RECONSTRUCTION?

Michael Johnson, PT, DSc, OCS, SCS;
Brett D. Owens, MD; and
Kenneth L. Cameron, PhD, MPH, ATC, CSCS

Chronic lateral ankle instability in athletes often results from either a single severe lateral ankle sprain or multiple less severe sprains over time. For athletes who perform cutting or multiplanar sports, the loss of stability in the lateral ankle complex can lead to a significant decrease in performance and/or loss in playing time and can even be career ending. Lateral ankle reconstruction is a common orthopedic surgical procedure for athletes who have chronic functional or mechanical instability. While many techniques have been reported and are used, the modified Bröstrom repair is the most commonly performed procedure, and this chapter focuses on the rehabilitation associated with this technique. This procedure is effective at restoring mechanical stability in the lateral ankle, and a sound rehabilitation program is critical for restoring functional stability following surgery.[1] The purpose of this chapter is to discuss key considerations during each phase of the rehabilitation process that will lead to optimal clinical outcomes and return to activity following lateral ankle reconstruction.

McKeon PO, Wikstrom EA, eds. *Quick Questions in Ankle Sprains: Expert Advice in Sports Medicine* (pp 191-197).
© 2015 SLACK Incorporated.

Initial Phase: 0 to 6 Weeks After Surgery

The primary goals of this phase are to protect the repair while preventing excessive scar tissue that can result in a "stiff" ankle. It is not uncommon for patients to be immobilized after surgery in a cast or some form of splint. The duration of immobilization is generally based on surgeon preference and can vary from 4 weeks of non-weight bearing in a cast to 1 to 2 weeks in a posterior splint with touch weight bearing. At the 3- to 4-week mark, weight bearing should be increased (as tolerated), and the patient should be put into a walking boot or Cam-Walker. By 6 weeks after surgery, the patient should be fully weight bearing but still wearing a protective splint or ankle brace. In this early phase, a lateral wedge may be inserted in the shoe/boot to further protect the repair as weight bearing is increased. These strategies can aid in limiting frontal plane (primarily inversion) motion so the repair can properly heal while allowing sagittal plane motion and preventing stiffness.

In addition to protecting the repair, emphasis at this time should be placed on initiating straight line or sagittal plane motion through supervised exercise and activities of daily living. Generally, athletes who require full sagittal plane range of motion (ie, gymnasts) will be immobilized for shorter periods of time than those in the general population.[1] Regaining ankle plantar flexion and dorsiflexion range of motion (ROM) in these patients is a priority, not only for general gait purposes but for higher level running and sprinting. It has been shown that a lack of dorsiflexion ROM can contribute to functional deficits and also lead to overuse problems at the knee.[2] These exercises put priority on regaining ROM but also allow the patient to start weight bearing, getting proprioceptive input to the ankle, and establishing a normal gait pattern. Keys to success and common exercises for this phase are listed in Table 37-1.

Phase 2: 7 to 12 Weeks After Surgery

Critical goals of this phase of rehabilitation include (1) obtaining full ankle eversion, plantar flexion, dorsiflexion, and 90% of the patient's inversion ROM and (2) having the patient perform a pain-free static hop. During this phase, the patient should also transition into normal footwear and may continue wearing some sort of lace-up or stirrup ankle brace while walking. Weight-bearing exercise should be a common theme in this phase. Keys to success and common exercises for this phase are listed in Table 37-2.

Weight-bearing stretching for the gastrocsoleus complex should be initiated. Evaluating ankle dorsiflexion ROM using a weight-bearing assessment method may be more functional during this rehabilitation phase (Figure 37-1).[3] Furthermore,

Table 37-1

Keys to Success and Common Exercises for Phase 1

Keys to Success for This Phase	Common Exercises for This Phase
Allow the repair to heal	Active ROM into dorsiflexion, plantar flexion, eversion, and inversion to neutral
Prevent excessive ankle stiffness (especially in plantar and dorsiflexion) through ROM exercises	Non-weight-bearing stretching of gastrocsoleus complex
Regain full weight-bearing status by 6 weeks after surgery	Seated wobbleboard exercises, weight shifting in the parallel bars; when surgical site is healed, pool rehabilitation is appropriate

Table 37-2

Keys to Success and Common Exercises for Phase 2

Keys to Success for This Phase	Common Exercises for This Phase
Weight-bearing stretching for full ankle dorsiflexion ROM	Cone exercises, carioca, marching, retrowalking on variable surface densities (pads, foam)
Incorporation of multidirection exercises to further challenge the balance and proprioceptive system	Total leg-strengthening exercises to incorporate the hip and core musculature
Focus on total leg strengthening to incorporate the proximal knee and hip musculature in the lower body kinetic chain	Jumps onto higher surfaces (box or platform) to initiate early plyometric exercises

weight-bearing dorsiflexion assessments have been linked to important clinical and patient-reported outcomes. Limitations in any of the primary ankle motions should be addressed by assisted or manual stretching. Ankle-specific and total leg strengthening as well as progressive proprioceptive and balance exercises should be performed in rehabilitation sessions and as part of a home program.

These exercises not only put more demand on the ankle in a protected environment but also start to incorporate the proximal/hip musculature as the patient begins to integrate the lower body kinetic chain into the rehabilitation process. At the close of this phase, the rehabilitation should reflect a more broad

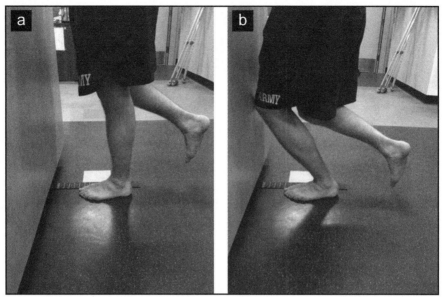

Figure 37-1. (A) Starting and (B) ending positions for the weight-bearing dorsi-flexion assessment.

lower-extremity approach and not be too "ankle specific." The "jump-up" exercises allow for early plyometric training without the added force and eccentric load that comes with landing or jumping off a higher surface.

Phase 3: 4 to 6 Months After Surgery

The critical goals of this rehabilitation phase for the patient include (1) being able to jog at the patient's own pace and distance without pain and (2) being able to hop for distance > 90% of the uninvolved side. This phase is generally when the patient will begin preparing for return to sport-type functions and demands on the ankle. A progressive jogging, strengthening, and plyometric program is a primary component of this phase. Straight-line exercises (running and jumping) would be initiated and then progress to more diagonal/dynamic jumping and cutting exercises. Keys to success and common exercises for this phase are listed in Table 37-3.

Examples of personalizing this rehabilitation phase could involve strengthening or proprioceptive exercises on a soft surface, or a low beam might be incorporated into rehabilitation for a gymnast in this phase. Sport-specific conditioning exercises should also be incorporated and progressed in this phase of rehabilitation as appropriate and tolerated.

Table 37-3

Keys to Success and Common Exercises for Phase 3

Keys to Success for This Phase	Common Exercises for This Phase
Being able to run at "game" speed in a straight line	A progressive running program focusing on the specific running demands for the athlete's sport
Being able to perform multidirectional and plyometric exercises aligned with the sports-specific demands of the athlete	Incorporation of higher or longer jumping and hopping exercises to progress the plyometric training components of the program
Personalizing rehabilitation exercises for the unique sport- or activity-specific demands of the athlete should be a primary focus	Replicating sport-specific demands to further prepare the athlete for return to sport as this phase progresses

Returning to Physical Activity and Sport

Key things to consider in making return-to-play decisions include (1) the amount of cutting or change of direction that occurs in the sport, (2) how well the patient can stabilize across the ankle when landing on the involved foot, and (3) if the patient continues to experience any mechanical or functional instability. Several functional tests have been developed and may be used to inform return-to-participation decisions. However, whether any test is appropriate first depends on how it aligns with the functional and physical demands of the athlete.

In general, tests that target agility may better represent the demands that are expected of the ankle. Additionally, these tests will stress the lateral ankle and will often bring about feelings of instability in the patient's ankle.[4] Although we have seen the value of hop tests as they pertain to the knee, shuttle runs may be more appropriate functional assessments of the ankle, requiring appropriate speed and the necessary agility of the ankle to complete the test.[4] Other tests to consider for return to play are the Y balance test-lower quarter (YBT-LQ) or the Star excursion balance test (SEBT).

The SEBT and YBT-LQ are dynamic tests that require strength, flexibility, and proprioception. The goal of the SEBT is to maintain a single-leg stance while reaching as far as possible with the contralateral leg in different directions (Figure 37-2). Plisky et al[5] and Gribble et al[6] have found that the SEBT and YBT-LQ are highly representative tests for the active population when looking at dynamic balance. Specifically, subjects with limited anterior reach on the SEBT,

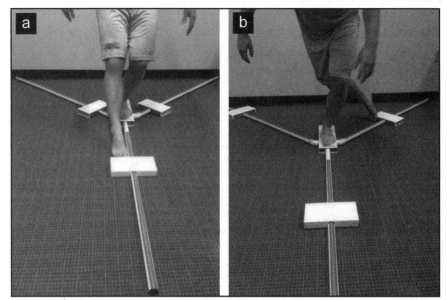

Figure 37-2. (A) Anterior reach for the Y balance test-lower quarter, which can identify deficits in dorsiflexion, and (B) medial reach, which assesses multiplanar stress on the ankle and lower extremity.

which requires good ankle dorsiflexion ROM, were more at risk for ankle injury. This demonstrates the utility of the SEBT and also the need for regaining ankle ROM following this surgery.[6]

Conclusion

Lateral ankle reconstruction is a common procedure in athletic populations. A rehabilitation program that addresses early ROM without compromising the repair and then incorporates a progressive functional strengthening program should allow the athlete to return to his or her previous level of function. Exercises that improve proprioception and balance and progress to sport-specific activities are also critical in the rehabilitation process for optimizing functional outcomes following surgery. Finally, using appropriate functional tests when assessing an athlete's ability to return to sport is important for ensuring that appropriate rehabilitation goals have been met and that the athlete is prepared for the physical demands of his or her sport.

References

1. Baxter DM. *The Foot and Ankle in Sport.* St. Louis, MO: Mosby; 1995.
2. Backman LJ, Danielson P. Low range of ankle dorsiflexion predisposes for patellar ten-dinopathy in junior elite basketball players: a 1-year prospective study. *Am J Sports Med.* 2011;39:2626-2633.
3. Konor MM, Morton S, Eckerson JM, Grindstaff TL. Reliability of three measures of ankle dor-siflexion range of motion. *Int J Sports Phys Ther.* 2012;7:279-287.
4. Caffrey E, Docherty CL, Schrader J, Klossner J. The ability of 4 single-limb hopping tests to detect functional performance deficits in individuals with functional ankle instability. *J Orthop Sports Phys Ther.* 2009;39:799-806.
5. Plisky PJ, Gorman PP, Butler RJ, et al. The reliability of an instrumented device for measuring components of the Star excursion balance test. *N Am J Sports Phys Ther.* 2009;4:92-99.
6. Gribble PA, Hertel J, Plisky P. Using the Star excursion balance test to assess dynamic pos-tural-control deficits and outcomes in lower extremity injury: a literature and systematic review. *J Athl Train.* 2012;47:339-357.

WHAT ARE THE SURGICAL AND REHABILITATIVE TREATMENT OPTIONS FOR AN ATHLETE WITH A COMBINED SYNDESMOTIC AND LATERAL ANKLE SPRAIN?

Kevin D. Phelps, MD and J. Kent Ellington, MD, MS

It is essential to maintain a high index of suspicion for syndesmotic injuries when treating athletes with ankle sprains. Syndesmotic injuries are reported to be present in anywhere from 1% to 18% of all ankle sprains and often go undiagnosed.[1] These injuries, also termed *high ankle sprains*, have been linked with longer recovery periods, greater functional impairment, and increased residual complaints 6 months after injury when compared to other types of ankle sprains.[2]

The most common mechanism for syndesmotic disruption involves an external rotation force at the ankle with the foot dorsiflexed and pronated, causing the rotational force of the talus to separate the fibula from the tibia. This initially results in tensioning and then rupture of the anterior inferior tibiofibular ligament. Continued external rotation leads to sequential disruption of the interosseous ligament, interosseous membrane, posterior inferior tibiofibular ligament, and transverse tibiofibular ligament. Clinically, the spectrum ranges anywhere from the more common ligamentous stretch injury to frank separation (diastasis) of the tibia from the fibula with associated bony or osteochondral injuries.

McKeon PO, Wikstrom EA, eds. *Quick Questions in Ankle Sprains: Expert Advice in Sports Medicine* (pp 199-202).
© 2015 SLACK Incorporated.

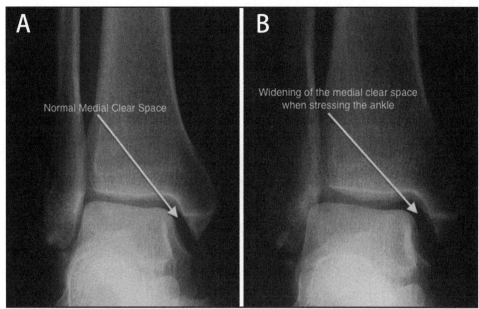

Figure 38-1. (A) Mortise view of the right ankle demonstrating no abnormalities. (B) Stress view of the same ankle demonstrating widening of the medial clear space when the ankle is stressed, indicating instability and associated syndesmosis injury.

During the initial evaluation, a thorough examination of the foot and ankle is necessary, noting any tenderness in the anterior lower leg between the tibia and the fibula. The distance that the tenderness extends proximally, termed the *tenderness length*, has been shown to have a positive correlation with injury severity and to be predictive of time lost from competition, with tenderness further proximally being predictive of a higher number of missed days.[3] Other provocative tests have been described and include the squeeze test, in which pain is reproduced at the ankle with medial-to-lateral compression of the leg at or slightly above the midcalf, and the external rotation test, in which the ankle is dorsiflexed while the foot is externally rotated, with pain indicating a positive test. Although highly specific, these tests have very low sensitivities, making it difficult to rely on them for the diagnosis of a syndesmotic injury. Initial radiographic evaluation should involve weight-bearing anteroposterior, mortise, and lateral views of the ankle.

The decision for surgical intervention is not always straightforward but is usually based on whether frank or latent (only detectable on stress or weight-bearing radiographs) diastasis of more than 2 mm is present. Without separation or instability with stress, patients can be placed in a cast or boot and allowed to bear weight immediately. Following boot or cast removal, the athlete then enters into a graduated therapy program such as that described later in this chapter. When no separation is detected between the tibia and fibula but widening of the medial clear space on stress radiographs is present (Figure 38-1), a conservative algorithm that

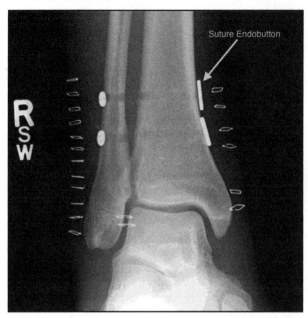

Suture Endobutton

Figure 38-2. Mortise view of a right ankle following endobutton suture fixation for a syndesmosis injury.

includes casting and non-weight bearing for 4 weeks followed by a walking cast for 2 to 3 weeks can be pursued. It is also reasonable to consider surgery for these types of injuries.

Surgical intervention is necessary when frank or latent diastasis of the syndesmosis is noted on weight-bearing or stress radiographs. Controversy exists in regards to the optimal surgical treatment of these types of injuries. The main discrepancies exist with regards to percutaneous vs open methods, screws vs suture endobutton fixation, and whether a plate should be placed on the fibula. Many advocate for either an open approach or ankle arthroscopy to directly inspect both the distal tibiofibular and ankle joint, as up to 28% of these injuries have associated talar dome osteochondral defects that should be addressed at the time of surgery.[4] Although one must be careful to protect the superficial peroneal nerve, open or arthroscopic evaluation also allows for careful positioning of the fibula within the incisura fibularis of the tibia during reduction of the syndesmosis.

Numerous studies have been performed to determine the most biomechanically sound construct for maintaining reduction of the syndesmosis. Two tricortical 3.5- or 4.5-mm screws, or the use of suture endobuttons (Figure 38-2), appear to provide the best fixation constructs. Regardless of the fixation method chosen, insertion should be within 2 cm of the tibiotalar joint line and at an angle of approximately 30 degrees from posterolateral to anteromedial. Bioabsorbable screws are gaining popularity, as they have a biomechanical profile similar to that of metallic screws and can eliminate the need for screw removal via a second procedure. Suture endobuttons provide a semirigid construct with dynamic stabilization and, in some studies, have been associated with a more rapid recovery and improved outcome scores.[5] Although advocated by some, the theoretical benefit from the addition of a plate as a means to enhance fixation and protect the fibula from future fracture has not been proven biomechanically. In the end, the specific method of fixation is likely less important than the accuracy of the reduction itself.

Postoperatively, patients are initially made non-weight bearing in a cast for several weeks, with specific time frames based on individual characteristics. If screws are placed for syndesmosis fixation, they are kept in place for a minimum of 6 to 8 weeks, with some advocating earliest consideration for removal at 3 months. Suture endobuttons do not require routine removal. Some treating physicians allow graduated weight bearing beginning at 6 weeks postoperatively with the screws in situ followed by an average time to removal of 8 to 10 weeks.

The optimal rehabilitation program for these injuries is currently unknown. Most current programs involve a minimum of 3 phases. The first phase is the acute phase, in which the primary goals are protection, pain control, and minimization of the inflammatory response. The second is a subacute phase, in which the focus is to restore mobility, strength, and function needed for basic activities. The last phase includes advanced training to prepare the athlete for return to sports. This phase emphasizes neuromuscular control, strength, and function in sport-specific tasks such as cutting, pivoting, and jumping.[6] Some recommend temporal guidelines for progression from phase 1 to 2, while others advocate for a criterion-based approach for progression. Patients should progress to phase 3 only once they are able to jog and hop repetitively on the previously injured leg without difficulty. Functional testing criteria are often used for return-to-sports decisions. These usually include activities such as forward hopping, vertical hopping, lateral hopping, sprinting, cutting, figure 8 drills, and backward pedaling. Athletes should be told up front that it may be 6 to 9 months before they are physically able to return to play at their previous functional level.

References

1. Rammelt S, Zwipp H, Grass R. Injuries to the distal tibiofibular syndesmosis: an evidence-based approach to acute and chronic lesions. *Foot Ankle Clin.* 2008;13:611-633, vii-viii.
2. Gerber JP, Williams GN, Scoville CR, Arciero RA, Taylor DC. Persistent disability associated with ankle sprains: a prospective examination of an athletic population. *Foot Ankle Int.* 1998;19:653-660.
3. Nussbaum ED, Hosea TM, Sieler SD, Incremona BR, Kessler DE. Prospective evaluation of syndesmotic ankle sprains without diastasis. *Am J Sports Med.* 2001;29:31-35.
4. Brown KW, Morrison WB, Schweitzer ME, Parellada JA, Nothnagel H. MRI findings associated with distal tibiofibular syndesmosis injury. *Am J Roentgenol.* 2004;182:131-136.
5. Anderson RB, Hunt KJ, McCormick JJ. Management of common sports-related injuries about the foot and ankle. *J Am Acad Orthop Surg.* 2010;18:546-556.
6. Williams GN, Jones MH, Amendola A. Syndesmotic ankle sprains in athletes. *Am J Sports Med.* 2007;35:1197-1207.

WHAT ARE THE SURGICAL AND REHABILITATIVE TREATMENT OPTIONS FOR AN ANKLE SPRAIN WITH A CHONDRAL DEFECT?

J. Kent Ellington, MD, MS and Matthew S. Wilson, MD

Osteochondral lesions of the talus involve injuries to the articular surface of the talar dome of the ankle joint and are a significant source of ankle morbidity. Over the course of the last 10 to 15 years, the phrase *osteochondral lesions of the talus* has been used to describe both osteochondritis dissecans and transchondral fractures of the talus. These injuries present a diagnostic and therapeutic challenge for the general practitioner, treating orthopedist, and rehabilitation professional, as articular cartilage (which covers 60% of the talus) is relatively avascular and thus has poor healing potential. The articulations between the talus and the tibial plafond and the lateral and medial facets of the talus with their respective malleoli form the ankle joint. The anatomy of the talus is such that it is the only bone through which the entire weight of the body is applied during locomotion, predisposing it to injury.

Etiology and Classification

Ankle sprains are an extremely common presenting complaint that the physician or rehabilitation specialist will encounter. In fact, one study demonstrated that

McKeon PO, Wikstrom EA, eds. *Quick Questions in Ankle Sprains: Expert Advice in Sports Medicine* (pp 203-207).

Table 39-1

Four Stages of Osteochondral Lesions of the Talus as Described by Berndt and Harty[2]

Stage 1	Small subchondral compression fracture
Stage 2	Partially detached osteochondral fragment
Stage 3	Completely detached osteochondral fragment without displacement
Stage 4	Completely detached osteochondral fragment with displacement

ankle injuries are the most common type of injury in 24 of 70 sports.[1] Multiple studies have demonstrated that 16% to 50% of acute ankle sprains will result in some form of articular cartilage injury, the most common of which is an inversion adduction mechanism that compromises the lateral ligament complex. Patients with ankle fractures have an even higher incidence of chondral injury. Proposed etiologies of ankle osteochondral lesions include local ischemia, acute trauma, chronic microtrauma, metabolic or endocrine factors, or genetic predisposition. Berndt and Harty[2] were the first to describe osteochondral lesions in the setting of trauma. Using a cadaveric model, they demonstrated that lateral talar lesions occurred in the setting of inversion and dorsiflexion of the ankle, while medial talar lesions were the result of inversion and plantar flexion. Flick and Gould validated this mechanism of injury by evaluating more than 500 patients and found that 98% of lateral talar lesions had a history of trauma, whereas only 70% of medial lesions were linked to trauma. Berndt and Harty[2] created a staging system (Table 39-1) based on radiographic findings during their review of the literature on transchondral fractures of the talus over a period of 100 years. Others have been developed, but the Berndt and Harty classification system remains the basis for staging osteochondral lesions and serves as the foundation for approach to treatment.

Clinical Presentation and Diagnosis

After an ankle sprain, patients generally experience 4 to 6 weeks of stiffness, swelling, and pain. In most cases, nonoperative management of icing, bracing, anti-inflammatory medications, proprioceptive training, and peroneal strengthening will lead to the resolution of symptoms. Those patients who present with refractory symptoms warrant a more detailed examination and a high clinical suspicion for an associated osteochondral lesion. Patients with an osteochondral lesion will often describe a deep, dull ache made worse with weightbearing and exercise but may also complain of mechanical symptoms such as locking or catching, which is consistent with a displaced cartilaginous fragment. Taga et al[4] evaluated 31 patients who complained of ongoing pain after an ankle sprain via arthroscopy and found that 89% of patients following an acute injury (6 to 8 weeks) and 95% of patients with chronic injuries (> 3 months) had an associated chondral injury.

Careful clinical examination is essential in these patients. A thorough examination of the hindfoot should be performed, including standing alignment, evaluating the ankle joint for effusion, and deep palpation of the anteromedial or anterolateral ankle joint for tenderness. Findings generally include the presence of an effusion and localized joint line tenderness. Range of motion should also be measured to determine any asymmetry relative to the contralateral side and to determine if this elicits mechanical symptoms. Ligamentous examination(s), inversion and eversion strength testing, and the anterior drawer test in both neutral and plantar flexion should also be completed.

Radiographs are critical in the evaluation of a patient who presents with trauma to the foot and ankle. Weightbearing anteroposterior, lateral, and mortise views are the standard initial studies ordered for patients with acute and/or long-standing ankle symptoms. Although initial radiographs are standard, they have a low sensitivity, an inability to assess the stability of the articular cartilage, and an inability to quantify the extent of an osteochondral lesion. In the setting of negative plain films and a high suspicion for an osteochondral lesion, magnetic resonance imaging (MRI) should be employed. MRI is considered the most sensitive diagnostic test for osteochondral lesions of the talus, as it can determine if the lesion is displaced and identify any other associated pathology. T2-weighted MRI will demonstrate intraosseous edema and hemorrhage and can also identify an unstable lesion which is depicted by a fluid rim of high signal intensity underneath the osteochondral lesion. Computed tomography can also be helpful in evaluating osteochondral lesions, specifically to identify cystic changes in the talus, and may alter treatment.

Treatment

Nonoperative management is the standard initial treatment for talar osteochondral lesions. An acutely displaced (> 2 mm) osteochondral lesion is the primary contraindication to initial nonoperative management. A period of 3 to 6 months of nonoperative management via cast immobilization or protected weight bearing in a walker boot, followed by progressive weight bearing and physical therapy, is recommended. Other experimental therapies exist (eg, hyaluronate and platelet-rich plasma injections, shock wave therapy), but the evidence remains preliminary. The success rate of nonoperative management for stable, nondisplaced lesions is less than 50%. Despite this, the available data support a trial of nonoperative management for all nondisplaced lesions.

Patients with refractory symptoms following a trial of conservative management or the presence of an advanced lesion (stage 3 or 4) should be offered surgical intervention. The treating surgeon has a continuously evolving armamentarium of both arthroscopic and open techniques at his or her disposal. Options include debridement, marrow stimulation, osteochondral allograft/autograft, and autologous chondrocyte implantation. Arthroscopy is used for small acute lesions and involves debridement of the unstable cartilage flap. Once a stable rim of articular cartilage is defined, marrow stimulation techniques are employed to promote reparative fibrocartilage. This has an average success rate of 85% to 90%.

Open procedures are recommended if initial arthroscopic procedures fail to provide relief, in the setting of large ostehochondral lesions (> 1.5 cm), and in those lesions that involve the shoulder of the talus—uncontained defects extending into the gutter. Osteochondral autograft is composed of hyaline cartilage and subchondral bone and can be harvested from the non-weight-bearing articular surface of the femoral condyle as well as the ipsilateral talus. Osteochondral allografts are also a source of osteoarticular material. Allografts are used in the setting of large defects or lesions of the shoulder of the talus that are difficult to treat with osteochondral autograft. The use of allograft eliminates donor site morbidity and is relatively unlimited for the treatment of larger lesions but increases disease-transmission risk, the long-term time interval for graft incorporation, and the rate of fragmentation and resorption. A third technique is autologous chondrocyte implantation (ACI). This is performed as an open procedure and involves the transplantation of cultured chondrocytes into an osteochondral lesion and is completed by covering the lesion with a periosteal patch that is sealed with fibrin glue. This technique requires 2 separate surgical procedures, the first to harvest the intact cartilage from the talus or the femoral condyle and the second involves reimplantation of the cultured chondrocytes. The early results of ACI appear promising with improved functional scores and high rates (> 80%) of return to full activity between 8 and 12 months.[5]

Conclusion

The size of the osteochondral lesion, the amount of displacement, and the chronicity of the patient's symptoms all play a critical role in the therapeutic algorithm of osteochondral lesions of the talus. The literature supports an initial trial of nonoperative management for small lesions without significant displacement. When nonoperative treatment fails, arthroscopy with debridement and marrow stimulation techniques are considered first-line treatments. Patients with lesions that have been untreated for longer than 4 to 6 months, are larger than 1 to 1.5 cm, or have failed arthroscopic treatment are candidates for osteochondral autograft/allograft or ACI.

References

1. Fong DT, Hong Y, Chan LK, Yung PS, Chan KM. A systematic review on ankle injury and ankle sprain in sports. *Sports Med.* 2007;37:73-94.
2. Berndt AL, Harty M. Transchondral fractures (osteochondritis dissecans) of the talus. *J Bone Joint Surg Am.* 1959;41:988-1020.
3. Easley ME, Latt LD, Santagelo JR, Merian-Genast M, Nunley JA. Osteochondral lesions of the talus. *J Am Acad Orthop Surg.* 2010;18:616-630.
4. Taga I, Shino K, Inoue M, et al. Articular cartilage lesions in ankles with lateral ligament injury. An arthroscopic study. *Am J Sports Med.* 1993;21:120-126.
5. McGahan PJ, Pinney SJ. Current concepts review: osteochondral lesions of the talus. *Foot Ankle Int.* 2010;31:90-101.

FINANCIAL DISCLOSURES

Dr. Brent L. Arnold has no financial or proprietary interest in the materials presented herein.

Dr. Javier Beltran has no financial or proprietary interest in the materials presented herein.

Dr. Chris M. Bleakley has no financial or proprietary interest in the materials presented herein.

Dr. Cathleen N. Brown has no financial or proprietary interest in the materials presented herein.

Dr. Joshua Burns has no financial or proprietary interest in the materials presented herein.

Dr. Kenneth L. Cameron has no financial or proprietary interest in the materials presented herein.

Dr. Brian Caulfield has no financial or proprietary interest in the materials presented herein.

Dr. Lisa Chinn has no financial or proprietary interest in the materials presented herein.

Dr. Mitchell L. Cordova has no financial or proprietary interest in the materials presented herein.

Dr. Eamonn Delahunt has no financial or proprietary interest in the materials presented herein.

Dr. Carrie Docherty has no financial or proprietary interest in the materials presented herein.

Cailbhe Doherty has no financial or proprietary interest in the materials presented herein.

Michael G. Dolan has no financial or proprietary interest in the materials presented herein.

Dr. Luke Donovan has no financial or proprietary interest in the materials presented herein.

Dr. Eric Eils has no financial or proprietary interest in the materials presented herein.

Dr. J. Kent Ellington has no financial or proprietary interest in the materials presented herein.

Dr. Todd A. Evans has no financial or proprietary interest in the materials presented herein.

Dr. Chad M. Ferguson has no financial or proprietary interest in the materials presented herein.

Dr. François Fourchet has no financial or proprietary interest in the materials presented herein.

Dr. Philip Glasgow has no financial or proprietary interest in the materials presented herein.

Dr. Phillip Gribble has no financial or proprietary interest in the materials presented herein.

Dr. Jay Hertel has no financial or proprietary interest in the materials presented herein.

Dr. Claire E. Hiller has no financial or proprietary interest in the materials presented herein.

Dr. Matthew C. Hoch has no financial or proprietary interest in the materials presented herein.

Dr. J. Ty Hopkins has no financial or proprietary interest in the materials presented herein.

Dr. Tricia Hubbard-Turner has no financial or proprietary interest in the materials presented herein.

Dr. Darren James has no financial or proprietary interest in the materials presented herein.

Michael Johnson has no financial or proprietary interest in the materials presented herein.

Dr. Thomas W. Kaminski has no financial or proprietary interest in the materials presented herein.

Jupil Ko has no financial or proprietary interest in the materials presented herein.

Dr. John E. Kovaleski has no financial or proprietary interest in the materials presented herein.

Dr. Tennyson Maliro has no financial or proprietary interest in the materials presented herein.

Dr. Carl G. Mattacola has no financial or proprietary interest in the materials presented herein.

Dr. Timothy A. McGuine has no financial or proprietary interest in the materials presented herein.

Dr. Patrick O. McKeon has no financial or proprietary interest in the materials presented herein.

Dr. Jennifer M. Medina McKeon has no financial or proprietary interest in the materials presented herein.

Eric Nussbaum has no financial or proprietary interest in the materials presented herein.

Dr. Brett D. Owens has no financial or proprietary interest in the materials presented herein.

Dr. Kevin D. Phelps has no financial or proprietary interest in the materials presented herein.

Thomas L. Pommering has no financial or proprietary interest in the materials presented herein.

Dr. Leah H. Portnow has no financial or proprietary interest in the materials presented herein.

Kelli Frye Pugh has no financial or proprietary interest in the materials presented herein.

Dr. Adam B. Rosen has no financial or proprietary interest in the materials presented herein.

Dr. Scott E. Ross has no financial or proprietary interest in the materials presented herein.

Helene Simpson has no financial or proprietary interest in the materials presented herein.

Dr. Kelli R. Snyder has no financial or proprietary interest in the materials presented herein.

Matthew Stewart has no financial or proprietary interest in the materials presented herein.

Dr. James C. Sullivan has no financial or proprietary interest in the materials presented herein.

Dr. Joseph Surace has no financial or proprietary interest in the materials presented herein.

Dr. Masafumi Terada has no financial or proprietary interest in the materials presented herein.

Dr. Jeffrey D. Tiemstra has no financial or proprietary interest in the materials presented herein.

Dr. Evert Verhagen is the developer of the smartphone application, "Ankle."

Dr. Bill Vicenzino has no financial or proprietary interest in the materials presented herein.

Dr. Brian R. Waterman has no financial or proprietary interest in the materials presented herein.

Caitlin Whale has no financial or proprietary interest in the materials presented herein.

Dr. Tine Willems has no financial or proprietary interest in the materials presented herein.

Dr. Erik A. Wikstrom has no financial or proprietary interest in the materials presented herein.

Dr. Matthew S. Wilson has no financial or proprietary interest in the materials presented herein.

INDEX